Palgrave Macmillan Studies in Family and Intimate Life

Series Editors
Graham Allan
Keele University
Keele, UK

Lynn Jamieson
University of Edinburgh
Edinburgh, UK

David H.J. Morgan
University of Manchester
Manchester, UK

'The Palgrave Macmillan Studies in Family and Intimate Life series is impressive and contemporary in its themes and approaches'—Professor Deborah Chambers, Newcastle University, UK, and author of *New Social Ties*.

The remit of the Palgrave Macmillan Studies in Family and Intimate Life series is to publish major texts, monographs and edited collections focusing broadly on the sociological exploration of intimate relationships and family organization. The series covers a wide range of topics such as partnership, marriage, parenting, domestic arrangements, kinship, demographic change, intergenerational ties, life course transitions, step-families, gay and lesbian relationships, lone-parent households, and also non-familial intimate relationships such as friendships and includes works by leading figures in the field, in the UK and internationally, and aims to contribute to continue publishing influential and prize-winning research.

More information about this series at
http://www.palgrave.com/gp/series/14676

Paulina Billett • Anne-Maree Sawyer

Infertility and Intimacy in an Online Community

palgrave
macmillan

Paulina Billett
La Trobe University
Melbourne, Australia

Anne-Maree Sawyer
La Trobe University
Melbourne, Australia

Palgrave Macmillan Studies in Family and Intimate Life
ISBN 978-1-137-44980-1   ISBN 978-1-137-44981-8   (eBook)
https://doi.org/10.1057/978-1-137-44981-8

Library of Congress Control Number: 2018953326

This Palgrave Macmillan imprint is published by the registered company Springer Nature Limited
The registered company address is: The Campus, 4 Crinan Street, London, N1 9XW, United Kingdom

Acknowledgements

To all the remarkable women who we met through this journey: without you, this book would have been impossible. Thank you for the trust you have placed in us to share your stories with the rest of the world. Your strength, courage and resilience are deeply inspiring.

This book is dedicated to you.

Contents

1

Introduction

Paulina Billett

Journey to the Other Side

I am sure many people are curious as to what drove us to write this book. Aside from a strong academic interest in the lives of women, there is also a deep personal motivation for us to undertake this task. In truth, we come from two very different places; one of us is childless by choice, while the other has battled with infertility since her early 30 having undergone several in vitro fertilisation (IVF) treatments and two miscarriages. Usually these two sides do not find much common ground, often regarding each other from across the "fertility trenches" with suspicious eyes. Yet, in reality, these two positions as childless women, in a society that venerates motherhood, share more commonalities than could have been expected.

From comparing our own stories, we learned that fertility and motherhood are neither a certainty nor a natural desire but, instead, a deeply

P. Billett (✉)
La Trobe University, Melbourne, Australia
e-mail: p.billett@latorbe.edu.au

© The Author(s) 2019
P. Billett, A.-M. Sawyer, *Infertility and Intimacy in an Online Community*,
Palgrave Macmillan Studies in Family and Intimate Life,
https://doi.org/10.1057/978-1-137-44981-8_1

1

personal struggle. We both found that the experience of not having children deeply affects the ways we see ourselves and how others see us. We
realised that often our childlessness comes as a bit of a shock to those who
wrongly assume that well-educated women in their 40s and 50s would
surely have had the good "sense" to reproduce. We have also come to
realise that the stereotype of woman's destiny equals motherhood is still a
strong narrative of western society and that the normative force of this
narrative has, to some extent, coloured much of our personal adult female
lives. We have often doubted our decisions and second guessed ourselves;
we have struggled with the labels placed on childless women and have at
times been deeply shocked by what others feel is their right to comment
about what is believed to be a very personal condition.

In my case, there were two main occurrences which triggered the desire
to write this book. The first was a good friend, who sought to comfort me
after my first devastating miscarriage by stating that I should not be worried as, after all, "smart women tend to have less children in the first
place"; the second was a well-meaning older student of mine who, in no
uncertain terms, told me that I should consider having kids now "as you
know dear you don't have forever to make these decisions".

Understandably both these assertions rocked me to the core. Suddenly
I began to see myself as others saw me, as somehow unnatural, defective
and perhaps a little selfish. This coupled with my own sense of disappointment and the inevitable insecurity, which unsuccessful IVF treatment and miscarriages seem to produce, got me thinking about how
infertility affects women at a personal level—how this disease profoundly
changes our biographies and sense of self at the deepest of levels. I began
paying closer attention to the experiences being described by my infertile
"sisters" on our online support group, and soon a pattern began to emerge.
Infertility is a life altering experience, one that changes us so deeply, that
even the safe arrival of children can never hope to erase. Furthermore, I
became deeply conscious that many of those dealing with infertility found
little comfort or understanding in "the real world" and instead found
solace with others also struggling in online support groups, forging deep
friendships that have spanned both the real and virtual worlds.

The stories which we relate in this book attest to this. By following the
journals and posts written by the women over a period of six years, we

relate the struggles faced in coming to terms with infertility. We describe the pain and frustration these women have felt at being unable to achieve what is commonly viewed as a woman's right. Yet these women are not victims, but instead show a capacity to overcome adversity, which is utterly spectacular. To this end, we also discuss the strategies they employ to survive in what they often consider to be the hostile fertile world.

Infertility and Its Impact on Sufferers

Infertility can be defined as "a disease of the reproductive system defined by the failure to achieve a clinical pregnancy after 12 months or more of regular unprotected sexual intercourse" (Zegers-Hochschild et al. 2009). This rather sterile, and fuss free medical definition for what may for many be a life altering experience, fails to describe the complex nature of the situation, or the experiences of those who live through it. While the impact of infertility is severe for a couple, it can be argued that for women, the burden of infertility is doubly hard to carry (Thompson 2002). Western constructions of femininity are closely tied to mothering, and women in most if not all cultures around the globe are defined through their reproductive capacity. In fact, most cultures assume that all women will want to have children, a desire which is believed to be biological in its origin (Inhorn and van Balen 2002).

Not surprisingly, most young women grow up with the expectation that one day they will find a suitable life partner and will become mothers; infertility is seldom if ever discussed as a possibility. Not surprisingly, the belief that motherhood is certain has resulted in sexually active women taking all manner of precautions not to fall pregnant. In fact, fertility is seen as so natural that even medical practitioners will not begin testing until a woman has tried to conceive for at least six to eight months (longer if she is under the magical age of 35) even when there may be reason for a couple's concern. As a result, the experience of being infertile in a society that venerates fertility is not an easy one. Women who want children but are unable to conceive or carry a pregnancy to term often feel confused, lost, purposeless and alone.

As can be seen, infertility is far from resembling its clinical description, but instead constitutes, what Giddens (1979) termed, a critical situation;

a major kind of disruptive experience which can severely affect a couple's, and in particular a woman's, biography. It constitutes a shift, which permeates every aspect of her life. For many women, their childlessness is seen as a personal failure, a failure of their body to engage in what they feel should be a natural process. As such, a number of stories recount the feelings of anger, sadness and frustration at their bodies' inability to conceive. Furthermore, infertility is also an intensively private matter that often spills out on to the public arena. Countless times, the women who shared their stories with us recounted in their posts and journals how society had little sympathy for those struggling with treatment. A number of women discussed how employers were largely unsympathetic to their needs, and the sense of "expert entitlement" felt by well-meaning individuals leading to the offering of (un) "helpful" advice on how to get pregnant. Finally, the struggle with infertility was made even harder by media stories which, while promoting motherhood as natural, paint the use of Assisted Reproductive Technology (ART) in a negative light. In fact, the demonising of ART has been so pervasive that in some countries the availability of treatment has been affected by these stories. For example, the news stories on Hollywood actress Nicole Kidman's use of IVF and a surrogate in 2011 changed Australian laws on surrogacy, almost completely destroying the ability of couples to make use of surrogates for pregnancy.

The intense feelings raised by the struggle with infertility, coupled with the strong public opinion prompted by the use of ART, has led many infertility sufferers to remain silent about their struggle. Yet the lack of input in this debate by those who are most vested in it, has contributed to a lack of recognition of infertility as a disease which places severe financial, physical and emotional burdens on suffers due to a lack of adequate support and response in government policy and medical care (Throsby 2004).

The Cost of Reproductive Technology

Infertility is a booming business. It is suggested that around 70 million couples are afflicted by infertility around the world with the numbers expected to increase by 5–10% annually (Brezina and Zhao 2012) making this a billion-dollar market. Infertility is most often addressed through

ART, a group of procedures "that involve the in vitro (outside the body) handling of human oocytes (eggs) and sperm or embryos for the purpose of establishing a pregnancy" (Macaldowie et al. 2013). There are a number of ARTs currently in the market. It could be argued that the main forms of ARTs take the form of[1]:

In vitro fertilisation (IVF): A procedure whereby an egg (or more than one egg) is retrieved from the body of a woman and combined with sperm outside the body to achieve fertilisation. If fertilisation is successful and the fertilised egg continues to develop to form an embryo, the embryo is subsequently transferred back into the uterus/fallopian tube of a woman with the aim of achieving a pregnancy. If many embryos develop, some of the surplus embryos may be frozen and used later.

Intracytoplasmic Sperm Injection (ICSI): An IVF technique where to achieve fertilisation a single sperm is injected directly into an egg.

Frozen Embryo Transfer (FET): Where an embryo that has been frozen (cryopreserved) is thawed and then transferred to the uterus/fallopian tube of a woman with the aim of achieving a pregnancy.

Gamete Intra-Fallopian Transfer (GIFT): A procedure where an egg (or more than one egg) retrieved from the body of a woman and sperm obtained from a male are both inserted back into the fallopian tube of a woman, with the aim to achieve fertilisation (and then pregnancy) within the body of the woman.

Assisted hatching: An IVF micromanipulation in which a small opening is made in the zona pellucida of an embryo to help the blastocyst emerge prior to implantation.

Intrauterine insemination (IUI): Entails the insertion of a catheter into the woman's uterus to deliver prepared sperm around the time of ovulation. However, according to a number of fertility treatment clinics, the success rate tends to be lower than other forms of ART.

Each patient's treatment may require the use of one or more of these procedures, making the treatment of patients through ART highly complex. In fact, patient choice in treatment is largely avoided; instead, doctors tend to make the decisions as to what level of intervention is required to give the patient "maximum" chance. Not surprisingly, the knowledge field of reproductive technology is jealously guarded, and not all doctors can practise as fertility specialists.

In Australia, as in much of the world, fertility specialists are required to undertake lengthy training as well as maintaining specialist registration to enable them to practise. Furthermore, the exorbitant costs associated with the science and technology behind ART has meant that rich conglomerates, in the guise of fertility clinics, have grown to dominate much of the ART industry including its research and development. The small number of ART service providers together with the increase in couples accessing treatment has aided the industry in becoming a billion-dollar venture, though academics and media reports often claim that success rates are over inflated (see for example Medew 2016; Deonandan et al. 2012) to the extent that in 2016 Australia's Consumer watchdog, the Australian Competition and Consumer Commission, launched an investigation into the presentation of success rates by Australian clinics after receiving complaints about potentially false or misleading claims from the Australian Health Practitioner Regulation Agency.

The controversies of the last few years, however, are nothing new. From its establishment, the science and history of ART has been highly contentious. ART spans over 30 years since the birth of the first "test tube baby", Louise Joy Brown, born in 1978 in England to Lesley and John Brown, after intervention from Doctors Robert Edwards and Patrick Steptoe. Her birth heralded a new era in reproduction, with couples unable to conceive finding new hope in the emerging technology. However, many individuals, and in particular church groups, vehemently opposed the creation of children via ART and felt that the technology represented a violation of natural order and God's law.

Since the birth of baby Louise, the use of ART to achieve pregnancy has become increasingly more commonplace with around 71,516 ART cycles initiated in 2013 in Australia and New Zealand alone (Macaldowie et al. 2013). However, the suspicion held by the public towards this technology has not altered since its introduction in the late 70s. IUI, IVF, GIFT, ICSI, donor sperm, egg and embryo adoption are among the many words which create the hurricane of responses to the experiences of a couple's infertility. This has been driven by two main concerns; the lack of clear global guidelines governing ethical standards for the ART industry and public perception of ARTs as dangerous. While the concerns held by the public seem to be similar around the globe, the responses to these concerns have varied substantially between countries. For example, Australia, New Zealand and the UK have addressed anxiety created by ART by developing strong regulatory legislation through government policy. This has included policing who can access ART, under what conditions egg and sperm donation is conducted and what ethical and safety precautions must be observed when storing or disposing of embryos (particularly embryos donated for research purposes). However, other countries such as the US (while having some regulation enshrined in legislation that is limited in scope) have left regulation largely in the hands of professional bodies. This has led to vast differences in reporting of success rates, collection of information on the use of donor gametes and most notably, the monitoring of the (un)ethical use of surrogates (Frith and Blyth 2014).

Few debates have affected the practices of the ART industry as much as the surrogacy debate. Surrogacy is "an arrangement in which a woman becomes pregnant and gives birth to a child for someone else" (Humbyrd 2009). This type of arrangement may or may not include the woman donating her eggs towards the pregnancy. Surrogacy is indeed a necessary piece of the puzzle for many couples. For women unable to conceive, or carry a pregnancy to term, (as well as gay couples) a surrogate may indeed be the only option left to them for forming their family. The debate surrounding surrogacy has been primarily driven by fear that surrogacy directly harms the surrogate mother; and, by its (perceived) harm of society (Peng 2013).

Harm to the surrogate mother has largely centred on issues of exploitation of underprivileged women (particularly) by wealthy western couples. Surrogates are often depicted as women with little education, income and very little personal security (Peng 2013) who are lured into surrogacy by the promise of increasing household income which may not otherwise be readily available to them. This depiction of the "vulnerable woman" together with the fact that surrogacy is a multimillion-dollar industry has created a situation whereby paid surrogacy has come to be seen as an immoral and exploitative practice, based on monetary coercion. Yet a number of studies have shown that this may not be the case and that, for many women, the drive to become a surrogate may arise from desires outside monetary motivations (Peng 2013).

The (perceived) harm to society is even more complex. Surrogacy challenges social norms regarding motherhood and family, as it is seen as "abnormal" for a mother to happily "handover" her child. Hence the behaviour of surrogates is often pathologised, seen as clear evidence of the disintegration of the family, the commodification of women's bodies and a violation of the child's right to know their "family". Not surprisingly, stances towards surrogacy vary greatly from country to country and in some cases, between states within the same nation. A small handful of countries, including Japan, Ireland and France have banned all types of surrogacy while in many parts of the world, including the UK, Australia, New Zealand and Hungary, only altruistic surrogacy is permitted, with commercial surrogacy carrying heavy penalties including jail time. Finally, nations such as Iran, Greece (though this is currently restricted to nationals) and the US (this differs from state to state) allow for commercial as well as altruistic surrogacy.

The large range of positions on surrogacy has created a number of issues for those attempting to access this service as well as for those attempting to regulate it. As we have noted, in much of the world, only altruistic surrogacy is acceptable, however, the legal and logistical constraints placed on the engagement of an altruistic surrogate are considerable. For example, in Australia, surrogacy laws are extremely complex. In many states and territories, it is illegal to advertise for a surrogate and agreements are not binding, which means that the surrogate (who is considered legally as the mother) can change her mind and choose to keep the child. In many states, where altruistic surrogacy is legal, only unpaid advertising can be undertaken, and under no circumstances can an individual residing in a state or territory where surrogacy is illegal engage in advertising in a 'legal state'. Potential surrogates must reside in States or Territories where surrogacy is legal. Finally, upon the child's birth, further legal steps (parenting orders or adoption) are required to transfer full custody to the intended parents.

New Zealand's laws on surrogacy, like Australia, also do not recognise surrogacy agreements as legally binding, and the surrogate is considered the mother until adoption arrangements are made. In the UK it is illegal to advertise for, or as, a surrogate and surrogacy agreements are not enforceable, presenting the same issues as the Australian and New Zealand examples. However, in the UK, the surrogate's husband is also considered to be the child's parent, further complicating the situations for those entering into an agreement, making surrogacy a highly stressful situation. What is more, the intended parents may not be the only ones to find the lack of enforceability problematic. Surrogates can and have found themselves in difficult situations whereby the future parents may choose to withdraw from the agreement, including after the child's birth. This has occurred in a handful of cases with the "baby Gammy" case the most public retranction to date.

The lack of certainty in altruistic arrangements may result in couples considering countries where surrogacy agreements are binding through the engagement of commercial surrogates. This is also true in countries where surrogacy of any kind is deemed illegal, leaving the couple with the only option of seeking a surrogate abroad. However, this is not without consequences. In most developed nations, such as the US, commercial surrogacy is extremely expensive. In most cases the couple will need to meet all legal and medical costs as well as pay the commercial surrogate an honorarium. Not surprisingly, the enormous economic expense has resulted in an increasing number of couples looking for surrogates in countries where monetary exchange rates are favourable. For example, a couple wishing to undertake a surrogate arrangement in India will need to pay around $12,000 per agreement, instead of an estimated $80,000 to over $1,000,000 per agreement in the US (Boyce 2013). What is more, while the US maintains a high level of control over surrogacy operations (at least in terms of medical and legal obligations) control of the process may be limited in more cost-effective operations such as those being run in India, leading to a number of cases of alleged exploitation of women involved in the surrogacy industry. In response to this, once popular surrogacy hotspots such as Thailand and India have moved to ban commercial surrogacy altogether, a move which has greatly impacted couples wishing to pursue surrogacy as well as the surrogates themselves.

Aside from the surrogacy debate, public antagonism towards the use of ART has been created by sensationalist media pieces depicting the use of ART as dangerous, experimental and unethical; for example, the much publicised cases of Nadya Suleman—nicknamed "octo" mum by global media outlets after the birth of her octuplets with the aid of ART—and the tragic story of Carlyn Savage who had another woman's embryo implanted after a fertility clinic's blunder. Each of these cases incensed public opinion and spawned an increase in demands for the regulation of ART services, with calls often couched in concern for patient care. These demands have included the introduction of a maximum dosage level for the administration of pharmaceuticals, the banning of "older" mothers accessing ART, banning use of surrogates for profit, a mandated maximum number of embryos transferred and the increased control of storage, use and disposal of embryos.

Why the Experiences of Women?

Some would argue that writing a book such as this, with its focus on women, risks universalising (gendered) differences in experiences of infertility. After all, these individuals would contend that not all those going through fertility treatment are women. Others may object that we are discussing a subject such as the desire to have a baby as a "woman's issue".

The reality is that even as women, our ability to speak about ourselves is constantly challenged. Second wave feminism was much criticised for its blindness towards the diversity of women's lived experiences which often saw the under-representation of voices outside white parameters. As a result, we, as women and feminists, are constantly challenged on the relevance of our ability to represent women's voices and on our desire to speak about women. As noted by Woodward and Woodward (2009):

> Speaking and writing as a woman in the academy has come to be seen as problematic in much the same way as the category woman, which has become subject to instability, questions and challenges. Even the statement 'speaking as a woman' seems oddly quaint, as it appears to be making universalising claims.

While challenges to the universality of women's voices and even to the conceptualisation of women as a category are conducted in (post) feminist's debates (indeed a worthwhile pursuit), we believe that the link between woman and motherhood and the romanticisation of this pairing in the narrative of the experiences of infertility warrants its conceptualisation as "women's experience". As such, while trying to move away from biological determinist arguments of women and motherhood, we are able to explore women's lived experiences and the challenges which fertility treatment presents that arise from the participants' position as women and whose identity is negotiated and created as part of the cultural and societal construction of what a woman is.

Others may object to our choosing solely to research the experiences of heterosexual women over a more diverse selection, which includes lesbian women, or the experiences of men. The reality is that the experiences of infertility are largely different for lesbian couples who face a separate set of challenges rooted in societal scepticism and prejudice. This is even more so for gay couples seeking to have child through ART. It may be due to this that online support sites such as Stronger Together tend to attract individuals of homogenous sexual preferences who can come together and share a deep understanding of the challenges fertility treatments present. This is not to say that we never encountered women in same sex couples on Stronger Together, but their participation was usually short lived. Our observation of these women's participation showed that, while they were made to feel welcome, the difference in the experiences of fertility treatment and, in particular, in their relationship with others and their partners saw them moving on in search of others who could share this aspect of their journey.

Our choice to omit men's voices from the discussion may be called out by some as negating the experiences of half of those who are undergoing this journey. However, we argue that this is warranted as the focus of fertility treatment is almost exclusively on women and their bodies. During the initial phases of testing, it is women's bodies that are first invaded. They are poked and prodded, with countless procedures aiming to ensure that their reproductive cycle and organs are within "acceptable" parameters. Men's testing usually begins and ends, in one sperm test which determines whether a male factor is present and what, if anything needs to be done about it. From there, it is predominantly, if not exclusively, women's bodies that are put under the microscope in the hopes that the battery of treatment will produce the much longed for result.

Further to this, as will be explored in Chap. 6, even when male factor is present, and men's bodies are more intensely focused upon during treatment, it is women who carry much of the burden. Not only are women the focus and recipients of testing and treatment, but also those we researched with often discussed the need to protect their partners from the pressures of treatment and the scrutiny of society. As a result, fertility treatment is largely a woman's domain as is the ensuing impact of treatment.

What is more, society almost exclusively "blames" women for their infertility. It is not unusual to see media "blame" pieces that focus on a woman's lack of judgement (usually insinuating promiscuity or selfishness on her part) which has led to this regrettable situation. Men seldom, if ever, appear in these media pieces, with their sexual or career choices never questioned within the larger popular discourse on fertility treatment.

For these reasons, we chose only to speak to women. We wanted to hear their stories and retell them in their own voices. As women, we wanted to speak about women, and the uniqueness of their journey as they navigate the roller-coaster of infertility.

A Feminist Approach to Infertility

Feminists have always focused on dismantling patriarchal power over society. Women's role in reproduction and the family are seen by most as the primary source of men's power over women. Reproduction and its corollary, motherhood, are a particularly problematic ground for feminists; women's lack of control over their own reproductive function is believed to enable inequality. The ascription of motherhood as a woman's ultimate role in life is believed to support the ideological acceptance of this inequality. It is not surprising that feminists have long advocated reproductive rights for women: the right to contraception and abortion being focal points for second and third wave feminist movements. Contraceptive devices such as the pill finally made it possible for women to separate sexuality from childbearing. The right to abortion, which is still denied to many, further expands on this. We know that the right to contraception and abortion increases women's chances of participating in education and employment, as well as having a positive impact on their reproductive health. Yet the family as a social institution continues to undermine the gains made by contraception. This is because families are not natural, but are social productions institutionalised in law. They serve to reproduce gender roles and sustain the unequal division of labour, constraining women's opportunities and freedoms in the wider society. This is not to say that we disagree with the right to form a family, rather, we wish to point out that the production of a family as an institutionalised force can affect the experiences and opportunities available to women.

The ideal of the family is entrenched in western heterosexual culture. The idea that somehow an individual's life progression should shift, as a river would, from the family of origin to the family of procreation has been heavily scrutinised by feminists. Most famously, second wave feminists such as Betty Friedan (1963) and Germaine Greer (1984) have examined this narrative, helping to lay bare the intricate systems of myth and reality which underpin it. Friedan, in her seminal work *The Feminine Mystique*, suggests that while the early part of the twentieth century saw women push towards equality, by the 1940s and 1950s the resurgence of the "happy house wife" as a source of feminine identity saw young women return to this traditional role (not that it was ever totally abandoned). By the 1960s however, the bubble had begun to burst, and many women had begun to yearn for "something more" (Friedan 1963). For many, being a wife, mother and housekeeper was simply not enough, and they yearned for the challenges of the workplace. However, the dominant ideology at the time was that women could not possibly be unhappy in this natural role, but that this situation was the result of "the old problem—education: more and more women had education, which naturally made them unhappy in their role as housewives" (Friedan 1963, p. 11). In short, motherhood was once again deemed the only proper role for women. This was again echoed by Jessie Bernard in her work, *Women, Wives, Mothers* (1975) in which she discusses how 1970s women were giving voice to their discontent with the ideal of "selfless motherhood".

Similarly, Germaine Greer in *Sex and Destiny* (Greer 1984) argues that while the West professes a deep love and desire for children, exhibiting a deep concern with fertility, procreation and the role of children and young people as the future, its very structure fosters the exact opposite. Children, according to Greer, are habitually ostracised from adult society and motherhood is largely managed by "outside parties" such as medical experts and teachers. This means that while women are constantly bombarded with messages that procreation and motherhood are a woman's ultimate goal, the reality is that for many, motherhood may be deeply disappointing.

With this in mind, it is not hard to see why second wave feminists have had such a contentious relationship with ART. The explosion of fertility treatments largely coincided with second wave feminism and its intense examination of women's roles, medicalisation of women's bodies and focus on reproductive rights. Liberal western feminists saw ART as a way in which women could gain further control over their reproductive rights (Thompson 2002). Radical feminists on the other hand saw it as evidence of further control of women's reproduction by men and thus as working against the interests of women (Denny 1994). With the battle lines drawn, feminists writing on the use of technology for reproduction grew. However, the voices and experiences of those undergoing treatment were often neglected in preference for purely theoretical approaches (Denny 1994). As a result, women undergoing fertility treatment were (and some may say continue to be) positioned as "powerless victims, who only use technology, but do not control it" (Denny 1994); thus the research largely failed to validate their lived experiences.

Even today, while society has come to terms with women who "want more", the underlying assumption is that eventually, we will all move towards motherhood. Unlike in the early and mid-twentieth century, where motherhood had been spoken of in terms of a woman's default position, women in the late twentieth and well into the twenty-first century speak of it in terms of a choice. Hardly a day goes by without a new blog appearing which touts the wonders and hardships of motherhood. Many of these blogs self-identify as "empowering" women with their writers seeming to suggest, that by openly sharing the "realities" of motherhood, they are re-writing old scripts and are consciously shifting from second wave arguments of motherhood as oppression (for an excellent discussion see O'Reilly 2010). The simple message of these blogs is that motherhood is the new "cool" and that to truly be a successful woman in the twenty-first century, you must juggle (but not too success-fully) a computer, an intimate partner, a household, a job (which may or may not be related to blogging) and a baby bottle. This ideal is further compounded by the endless stories abounding in the online world and self-help collections, which minutely detail women's experiences of infer-tility and their "inevitable" success with ART.

It is thus unsurprising that even to this day most individuals would see family creation as a natural given; after all, an outcome where family is desired but not achieved is not only unspoken but almost unimaginable in our current cultural discourse. As a result, when a couple fails to make this expected transition, it is only to be expected that much confusion and sorrow should result, after all, even when the question of mother-hood has become one of "choice", the result—motherhood—remains the same. The lack of public discussion surrounding the inability to conceive or the impact that the loss of motherhood has on infertile women has meant that those undergoing ART often find little consolation or under-standing from fertile others.

While we do not ascribe to motherhood as a natural desire, we do sup-port the stance that infertility is a life-changing experience, which consti-tutes a critical situation for the majority of women diagnosed with this disease. We advocate an understanding of motherhood and parenting which moves beyond simply a question of oppression or simple choice and instead choose to see it as highly complex part of the larger identity puzzle; after all, motherhood and femininity are heavily intertwined in patriarchal society, making it hard for any woman to escape the confines of this label. In this, we align ourselves with early radical feminist writers such as Adrianne Rich (1977) who saw the label of motherhood, rather than parenting itself, as the source of patriarchal oppression which distorts women's experiences. As such, what we aim to examine are women's emo-tional landscapes as they navigate infertility and face the inability to par-ent, rather than women's response to motherhood. We would argue that feminists have too often failed to acknowledge the deep emotional impact the loss of motherhood can have on women. Simply hiding our heads under the proverbial blanket and not wishing to acknowledge this is non-sensical and, instead, we advocate an understanding of infertility and ART which considers the impact of infertility on women's lives and identities.

As a result, it is our hope that this book adds to the body of evidence which has at its heart "a sociology which is in the interest of women rather than only about women" (Acker et al. 1983, p. 424) and which provides a better understanding of how women's everyday experiences are produced within social contexts and structures. By using a woman-centred approach which focuses on the women's narration of their day to day struggle through the stories contained in their journals, together with posts made to their support group, we seek to demonstrate how women may be empowered by engaging with others online to tell their stories, share in their knowledge, sorrows and successes and find much needed understanding during this difficult period in their lives. In short, we wish to position the women away from the commonly attributed "victim" label and instead we demonstrate how they actively engage in decisions relating to their treatment, including its cessation, and as producers of their own biographies.

Re-imagining Community for the Online World

Where communities had previously focused on corporeal, tangible entities such as the neighbourhood or church group, the nature of sociality as it began to unfold online required a rethinking of what it meant to belong. Virtual communities, due to their lack of face-to-face interaction and extraterritoriality cannot be understood in the traditional sense (Blackshaw 2010). Traditional community requires physical copresence as well as continual interaction for familiarity to form (think for example of local community groups), allowing strong ties to form between individuals that can be accessed in times of need. Online communities however do not require physical interaction between individuals or even repeated interaction (though our research shows that members who maintained a regular presence in Stronger Together reported a stronger sense of community belonging). These communities also see individuals drop in and out depending on their need, (e.g. some members only used the site to vent, or to ask questions related to treatment). Theorists, such as Castells (Castells 2001) have argued that a shift has taken place in how we communicate with others, leading to the "privatization of sociability" (128).

Consequently, definitions of community require reconceptualisation away from geographical face-to-face copresence towards a more affective experience, which is highly personalised. In this context, a virtual or online community is defined as "groups of people with common interests and practices that communicate regularly and for some duration in an organised way over the internet through a common location or mechanism" (Ridings et al. 2002, p. 273).

In this sense, groups such as Stronger Together are online communities formed out of particular needs. These groups foster communities which allow for a range of forms of participation, from the stable member who may visit the site several times a day to the "lurker" who browses information posted by others. This allows the women to shift their identities from their offline selves and instead attend to an aspect of their identity: the infertile individual, who is usually hidden from wider society (for a more in-depth discussion see Chaps. 4 and 5).

As a result, the women in Stronger Together, as in many other online groups, can explore emotional aspects of their journey, such as anger, sorrow and hope with a community of others who, while not known physically, are best placed to understand their unique situations.

Offline Lives, Online Worlds

Online support groups such as Stronger Together have been found by researches to be valuable sources of emotional support and self-empowerment (Barak et al. 2008). Reaching out to a support group is often done due to a desire to belong to an entity which is composed of individuals who share similar issues and who may provide understanding, often lacking in offline interactions. As we have discussed previously in this introduction, and will expand on in subsequent chapters, women journeying through the gauntlet of fertility treatment can often feel isolated and misunderstood by others, and this sometimes results in choosing to breakaway from typical support structures such as friends and family. The online environment, built to accommodate a plethora of ideas, provides a safe environment in which the women are able to come together and discuss their journeys and, crucially, it provides a refuge from the onslaught of the fertile world.

An important feature of websites such as Stronger Together is their anonymity. The anonymity afforded by the internet can have a disinhibiting effect (see Chaps. 2 and 3) which allows those participating to express opinions which they may otherwise keep hidden from others. This allowed support group participants a space to "vent" feelings, such as jealousy, which they felt may not be supported in the offline world. As we describe more fully throughout the book, unsupportive behaviours and attitudes were often a source of angst for the women, and "venting" provided a safe outlet through which to express anger and resentment. Furthermore, through their journeys, women often expressed the need to simply talk about their experiences of infertility and treatment with others who they felt could understand their perspective. Having a safe space in which to discuss treatment, ask for advice, express disappointment or just muse without the fear of being judged, was an important resource gained in the online experience.

It was the sharing of these intense feelings, which also made the relationships developed online all the more significant. While relationships online are often discussed in academic literature as being less "real" than offline interactions, a growing body of evidence suggests that, at least for those needing support, online relationships can become as important as their offline equivalents. This was certainly the case for the women of Stronger Together, whose offline relationships had frequently been damaged by their experiences of infertility. As we discuss throughout this book, women facing infertility often isolate themselves from others as a self-protection mechanism. The ability to forge friendships online allowed these women to regain much needed support and helped to create a stronger sense of identity outside typical feminine parameters.

What is more, online friendships did not always remain contained within the confines of the online environment, but many moved into the offline world. During our time researching, we became aware that several women met offline during their journeys. Those in geographic proximity sometimes met informally and strong friendships formed. Furthermore, on occasion, results of treatment were delivered by Stronger Together friends to the rest of the online community, rather than by the individuals themselves. This was particularly true of birth announcements, which were often announced by friends after receiving phone calls. This suggests to us that these friendships are more than short term opportunistic networking but, in fact, present a form of intimacy that transcends cyber space.

About the Study

As we have briefly discussed in earlier sections of this introduction, what is sadly neglected amidst the cacophony of voices raised in the infertility debates are the experiences of those struggling with this disease. In this book, we have attempted to address this by allowing women to tell us, through their journals and posts, about their journeys through the labyrinth of infertility and fertility treatment. This book discusses the experiences of 24 women who underwent fertility treatment in the period between 2011 and 2017. After the project cleared the University Ethics Committee (Ethics Application Number 2044–14), a post was placed on the main discussion board of the Stronger Together website, inviting women into the study. The women self-selected into the study by taking a short survey and consenting to allow use of their journals (participants could manually lock any entries they did not wish us to use by switching those entries from viewed by public or friend to "private").

Those choosing to participate in the study were referred to an online survey which sought to gather background data about the women's lives, age, income and educational level, and the type, length and cost of fertility treatment. What we found was that these women were aged between 26 and 45, with the average being 32 years of age. On average, they had been trying to conceive for at least two years, with three women reporting their journey lasting over 10 years. The majority were well educated, possessing a university degree or higher qualification. Most also engaged in professional or para professional employment and all were involved in heterosexual relationships. On average, these women had spent at least 12 months undergoing fertility treatment at a cost of around $15,000 to $30,000 at the start of this research as well as several of them undertaking complementary fertility therapies (such as acupuncture and Chinese herbs).

In this book, we examine a number of journals and discussion board posts contributed to Stronger Together over a period of six years. In total, eight journals where selected for close thematic and narrative analysis (Creswell 2013; Riessman 2001; Silverman 2010). We developed a detailed set of codes (see Appendix A) through which to shape our analysis, and structure each chapter. The choice of journal was largely driven by the level at which the women were willing to share their stories with us and the wider public, with some women being happy for us to read their journals but not for their content to be published, while a range of posts to open access discussion boards were chosen to supplement and compare the experiences described in the women's journals. The choice of posts was made by selecting those that used key words describing the women's experiences; for example, when a journal described issues with partners, posts which included words such as "help", and "DH" (Dear Husband) were examined for comparison (see Appendix B for a list of commonly used abbreviations on the Stronger Together site). Similarly, if women spoke of a particular form of treatment and their experience of it, a search for posts about this particular treatment were sought. Our rationale for adopting this approach was due to our belief that because these posts and journals were self-determined, rather than driven by the researcher's interests, hypotheses or questions, they allowed us to get closer to the women's actual experiences. While our study relied on unobtrusive research methods, we acknowledge that the posts the women made to one another were shaped by the very particular (narrative) environment of Stronger Together, and that our analysis of their words was unavoidably influenced by our respective positions as female academics with very particular research and personal interests (Greene 2014). Finally, even though participants in Stronger Together chose an online name unrelated to their "real" offline one, these we felt may still lead to potential identification of participants via a web search. For this reason, new pseudonyms were given to each participant to ensure privacy and protect their identities.

Stronger Together

As a platform, Stronger Together can be classified as an open online space which provides its members with a range of opportunities to network with others. Through the platform, participants can add or respond to messages on the infertility forum or can add journal entries which can be set to a range of access levels, from personal access only, friends only to public access. While Stronger Together is not specifically geared to be an infertility support site, and in fact, the infertility discussion forum is one of over 500 such forums provided by Stronger Together, its infertility forum is well populated—boasting over 1000 individual members. Many of these members also belong to other Stronger Together groups, allowing Stronger Together participants to manage a range of issues simultaneously. This creates a holistic experience for its participants. Members of the infertility group also followed this pattern, with a proportion of its membership also engaging in forums that related to their specific conditions, such as endometriosis, Polycystic Ovarian Syndrome (PCOS), secondary infertility, adoption, miscarriage and still birth support groups among many others.

The rise of fertility therapy in the mid-seventies saw the creation of support groups for women dealing specifically with the complexity of infertility and its treatment. The first body advocating for infertile couples was RESOLVE: The National Infertility Association established in 1974 in the US. It was not until much later, in fact the beginning of the twenty-first century, that other national networks such as Access Australia registered in May of 2000 and Fertility Network UK (formerly *Infertility Network UK*) registered in England and Wales in 2003 and in Scotland in 2008. Each of these groups advocates for individuals struggling with infertility as well as disseminating information and providing face-to-face support groups.

However, membership of these networks is not straightforward. Each of these groups have hurdles to membership, with some requiring medical diagnosis before "admittance" while others also require payment of a membership fee. Requirements of payments and or medical diagnosis effectively impedes access for women who may not have met the medically imposed prerequisite time limit for testing (usually 18 months for a woman under the age of 35), or have the economic resources to access medical care or, as in the case of ACCESS, the ability and/or desire to pay the yearly fee on top of what can be an already expensive medical diagnosis and treatment. As a result, while we acknowledge the work of these bodies in advocating for those faced with infertility, we believe that their reach is mitigated by their formal requirements. It comes as little surprise that individuals are moving away from these traditional advocacy-centred groups and instead opting for the more flexible online support group. Online support groups do not require payment of fees or proof of diagnosis, meaning that individuals can engage much earlier in their infertility journey as well as "sample" a range of support groups, even before a diagnosis is made.

The Voice Behind the Mask

We believe that simply producing "disembodied" narratives is counterproductive when trying to bring the voices and experiences of women to the fore. For this reason, we would like to take the time to give some background to these unique accounts. To do this without violating the women's right to privacy, we have chosen to present their stories as part of a larger narrative by only selecting excerpts from their accounts to highlight the common issues which the women faced. This will allow the reader to gain a sense of their experience and, as we have come to see, to understand that the impact of infertility, far from being a single individual's experience, is a shared experience which shapes women in a number of ways.

While infertility is experienced at an individual level, and each woman's journey is different, the stories the women told through their journals and post spoke loudly of the collective experiences of infertile women. Each and every one of these women identified as infertile, whether or not the infertility was due to female or male factor or the more confounding category of unexplained infertility. For each of these women, regardless of which diagnosis they had received, their feelings of sadness, turmoil and isolation were very similar, suggesting that the emotions experienced during this journey were highly complex and stemmed from more than just a diagnosis. Most of these stories spoke of feelings of isolation from "fertile" society due to lack of empathy and understanding shown by others, leading to their choice to find support, comfort and understanding in the online world. For many, Stronger Together became a place in which to "vent" to others in a safe environment, a source of encouragement when difficult decisions needed to be made, and as a sounding board for their ideas and emotions.

Most of these women's accounts also discussed the difficulties faced in treatment, including their resentment at medical practitioners' focus on women's bodies in ART, as well as the negative impact this treatment had on their own mental, physical and emotional health and their economic wellbeing. By the time we undertook this research, a number of them had seen or had considered seeing more than one doctor. Most had at some point considered cessation of treatment, even for short periods of time. This was usually precipitated when patient care and empathy were felt to be lacking, or after unsuccessful treatment cycles and was often seen as a way of taking charge and regaining some control over their own lives.

Those who shared their stories with us struggled intensely with being labelled as infertile and often mused about what this meant in terms of their "femininity". A number of them described their bodies as "broken" and as time progressed became intensely disheartened by the process, particularly when the elation of seemingly successful treatment turned into heartbreaking miscarriage. Yet each and every one of these women did not see herself as a victim, rather, they saw their condition as a challenge to be resolved. For the majority, their struggle ended in "success" with a number of pregnancies and some adoptions occurring over the course of our research. Others have continued to struggle in their infertility journey. A further small number chose to end treatment and found varying degrees of comfort in this decision.

Shape of the Book

In this book, we have endeavoured to explore the impact of infertility on women's sense of identity and the ways in which the online world provides a place in which they can find comfort and support. Through the chapters we examine the women's stories, teasing out common themes and narratives in their struggle with infertility. We also illustrate our emerging observations of a phenomenon we named as the "triangulation" of the women's key relationships and intimacies in the setting of online support. Specifically, the women seemed to see themselves and their alliances, across online and offline worlds, through three intersecting nodes: online friendships; family, friends and work colleagues; and, their spousal partners. These nodes provided reference points for identity construction and also for a re-grouping of key intimacies, often in terms of an emotional prioritisation of online friends in the context of their struggles with infertility.

In The Changing Face of Society—Intimacy and Support in the Online World, we situate the proliferation of online support groups (OSGs) socially and historically, in relation to such developments as the rise of therapy culture. It provides an overview of the key features of health-related OSG participation, utilising recent studies from clinical/ health sciences and related insights from our participants. The chapter also reports on key debates in the research literature on OSGs, and outlines our contribution to the sociological study of infertility and online support. By approaching the "Stronger Together" OSG as a very particular narrative environment, we show how broader cultural narratives of self and infertility are inscribed in participants' online exchanges.

Finding Support in the Online World overviews the first node of the relationship triangle: online friends. In this chapter, we begin with an overview of the changes the concept of intimacy has undergone over the last 20 years, particularly in the light of challenges posed since the inception of the world wide web in the last decade of the twentieth century and the creation of online communities such as Stronger Together. We explore the use which the women make of the OSG environment and overview the benefits of OSGs for their users. We also outline the issues of copresence and anonymity and, finally, consider why some of these relationships moved into the offline world.

A Glance in the Mirror Women's Reflections on Their Emotions, Bodies and Selves focuses on the women's accounts of their selves, emotions and bodies in the online space. Specifically, we examine their language of selfhood and the frameworks they used to make sense of, and re-craft, their own and fellow members' stories as they navigated the "roller-coaster ride" of infertility. Through close readings of their posts, we show how participants were encouraged to "emplot" their experiences in specific ways. Individualised discourses of "positive thinking" and "working" on the self to enhance one's chances of falling pregnant were the dominant narrative resources deployed in online interactions. Significantly, several women "spoke back" to these discourses, questioning their utility, particularly after multiple failed treatments—a position not reinforced by other participants. In this context, we speculate on the lack of culturally prescribed narratives to guide these women into the future.

In Relationships in a Fertile World: Negotiating Alliances and the "Pregnant Other" we examine the destabilisation of key relationships in the women's lives in the context of infertility. Focusing on relationships with family, friends and work colleagues—the second node of the triangular relationship structure—we analyse the way they managed their emotions in encounters with these significant others, particularly with "pregnant others" towards whom they often felt ambivalence and anger. These unwelcome feelings were much maligned by the women themselves, as they struggled for emotional regulation.

In partnering the Infertile: The Impact of Infertility on Women's Spousal Relationships we explore the third node of the relationship triangle and examine the impact of the infertility journey on the couple's relationship. We begin by examining the challenges faced by couples from their inability to conceive. We pay attention to the couple's relationship and the destabilising impact of infertility. We examine how women navigate differences in responses by their partners to the infertility journey and the deep sense of abandonment women feel when their partners' reactions are not in line with their own. We move on to discuss the strategies which these women employ to re-stabilise their relationships and, finally, we turn our attention to the strategy of "partner protection" and its impact on the women's journey.

Finally, in Looking Back, Moving Forward we circle back to the main issues covered in the book and postulate on the future, particularly considering the rapid increase in internet-based modes of support, intimacy and identity creation. This chapter invites the reader to consider infertility in its socio-cultural context, to examine aspects of society that affect the experiences of those suffering from infertility. We examine once again relationships in the infertile world and the refuge that OSGs provide for those dealing with life-changing situations such as infertility. Lastly, we put forward some suggestions for practitioners who routinely work with those undergoing the infertility journey.

Note

1. Definitions derived from Zegers-Hochschild et al. (2009), Macaldowie et al. (2013) and The Reproductive Technology Council website.

References

Acker, J., Barry, K., & Joke, E. (1983). Objectivity and Truth: Problems in Doing Feminist Research. *Women's Studies International Forum, 6*(4), 423–435.

Barak, A., Boniel-Nissim, M., & Suler, J. (2008). Fostering Empowerment in Online Support Groups. *Computers in Human Behavior, 24*(5), 1867–1883.

Blackshaw, T. (2010). *Key Concepts in Community Studies*. London: Sage Publications.

Boyce, A. K. (2013). Protecting the Voiceless: Rights of the Child in Transnational Surrogacy Agreements. *Suffolk Transnational Law Review, 36*(3), 650–670.

Brezina, P., & Zhao, Y. (2012). The Ethical, Legal, and Social Issues Impacted by Modern Assisted Reproductive Technologies. *Obstetrics and Gynecology International*, Article ID 686253, 1–7.

Castells, M. (2001). *The Internet Galaxy: Reflections on the Internet, Business and Society*. New York: Oxford University Press.

Creswell, J. (2013). *Qualitative Inquiry & Research Design: Choosing Among Five Approaches*. Thousand Oaks: Sage.

Denny, E. (1994). Liberation or Oppression? Radical Feminism and In Vitro Fertilisation. *Sociology of Health & Illness, 16*(1), 62–80.

Deonandan, R., Green, S., & van Beinum, A. (2012). Ethical Concerns for Maternal Surrogacy and Reproductive Tourism. *Journal of Medical Ethics, 38*(12), 742–745.

Friedan, B. (1963). *The Feminine Mystique*. New York: W.W. Norton and Co.

Frith, L., & Blyth, E. (2014). Assisted Reproductive Technology in the USA: Is More Regulation Needed? *Reproductive Biomedicine Online, 29*(4), 516–523.

Giddens, A. (1979). *Central Problems in Social Theory*. London: Macmillan.

Greene, M. J. (2014). On the Inside Looking In: Methodological Insights and Challenges in Conducting Qualitative Insider Research. *The Qualitative Report, 19*(29), 1–13.

Greer, G. (1984). *Sex and Destiny: The Politics of Human Fertility.* New York: Harper and Row.

Humbyrd, C. (2009). Fair Trade International Surrogacy. *Bioethics, 9*(3), 111–118.

Inhorn, M., & van Balen, F. (2002). *Infertility Around the Globe: New Thinking on Childlessness, Gender, and Reproductive Technologies.* Berkeley: University of California Press.

Macaldowie, A., Lee, E., & Chambers, G. M. (2013). *Assisted Reproductive Technology in Australia and New Zealand 2013.* National Perinatal Epidemiology and Statistics Unit, the University of New South Wales. Retrieved from https://npesu.unsw.edu.au/sites/default/files/npesu/data_collection/Assisted%20reproductive%20technology%20in%20Australia%20and%20New%20Zealand%202013.pdf.

Medew, J. (2016, November 14). IVF Clinics Caught Making False and Misleading Claims About Success Rates. *The Age.* Retrieved from http://www.theage.com.au/victoria/ivf-clinics-caught-making-false-and-misleading-claims-about-success-rates-20161114-gsooix.html.

O'Reilly, A. (2010). *Twenty-First-Century Motherhood: Experience, Identity, Policy, Agency.* New York: Columbia University Press.

Peng, L. (2013). Surrogate Mothers: An Exploration of the Empirical and the Normative. *American University Journal of Gender, Social Policy and Law, 21*(3), 555–582.

Rich, A. (1977). *Of Woman Born: Motherhood as Institution.* London: Virago.

Ridings, C., Gefen, D., & Arinze, B. (2002). Some Antecedents and Effects of Trust in Virtual Communities. *Journal of Strategic Information Systems, 11*(3), 271–295.

Riessman, C. K. (2001). Personal Troubles as Social Issues: A Narrative of Infertility in Context. In I. Shaw & N. Gould (Eds.), *Qualitative Research in Social Work* (pp. 73–83). London: Sage.

Silverman, D. (2010). *Doing Qualitative Research.* London: Sage.

Thompson, C. M. (2002). *Fertile Ground: Feminists Theorize Infertility.* In M. Inhorn & F. van Balen (Eds.), *Infertility Around the Globe: New Thinking on Childlessness, Gender, and Reproductive Technologies* (pp. 52–78). California: University of California Press.

Throsby, K. (2004). *When IVF Fails: Feminism, Infertility and the Negotiation of Normality.* Hampshire: Palgrave Macmillan.

Woodward, K., & Woodward, S. (2009). *Why Feminism Still Matters: Feminism Lost and Found*. Basingstoke; New York: Palgrave Macmillan.

Zegers-Hochschild, F., Adamson, G. D., de Mouzon, J., Ishihara, O., Mansour, R., Nygren, K., et al. (2009). International Committee for Monitoring Assisted Reproductive Technology (ICMART) and the World Health Organization (WHO) Revised Glossary of ART Terminology. *Fertility and Sterility, 92*(5), 1520–1524.

2

The Changing Face of Society: Intimacy and Support in the Online World

Anne-Maree Sawyer

Journalling is "like a form of absolution for me." (Stronger Together participant)
"ST is a great place for support. Some of the greatest help I received was from this site. Knowing that I was not alone or crazy on this IF journey was life changing." (Stronger Together participant)

Introduction

Since the late twentieth century, the rise of the internet and online support groups (Osgs) has revolutionised the way individuals obtain health information and support (Mo and Coulson 2014, p. 984). This chapter situates the phenomenon of Osgs socially and historically, in relation to the rise of therapy culture and other developments. It provides an overview of the key features of health-related OSG participation, utilising

A.-M. Sawyer (✉)
La Trobe University, Melbourne, Australia
e-mail: a.sawyer@latrobe.edu.au

© The Author(s) 2019   **29**
P. Billett, A.-M. Sawyer, *Infertility and Intimacy in an Online Community*,
Palgrave Macmillan Studies in Family and Intimate Life,
https://doi.org/10.1057/978-1-137-44981-8_2

recent studies from clinical/health sciences and pertinent insights from our participants, and outlines our particular contribution to the sociological study of infertility and online support. By approaching the Stronger Together OSG as a very particular narrative environment, we aim to show throughout this book how broader cultural narratives of self, infertility and motherhood are inscribed in participants' online exchanges.

Over the past two decades, OSGs dedicated to specific forms of distress have proliferated to such an extent as to constitute a "mass social phenomenon" (Barak et al. 2008, p. 1868; see Chung 2013; Slauson-Blevins et al. 2013; Tanis 2007). These groups encompass an extensive and growing range of distress topics. Groups for sufferers of asthma, breast cancer, prostate cancer, depression, social phobia, fibromyalgia, chronic fatigue, multiple chemical sensitivity, HIV/AIDS, and infertility, along with victims/survivors of rape and domestic violence, smokers who are trying to quit and children whose parents have Alzheimer's Disease are but a small sample of these topics (see Barak et al. 2008, p. 1868; Tanis 2007). In an early large-scale study of face-to-face and online support groups representing 20 illnesses, Davison, Pennebaker and Dickerson (2000, p. 213) found that support seeking was closely related to the "interpersonal consequences of illness". Conditions experienced as embarrassing, stigmatising, or disfiguring, and as "less responsive to purely medical care", were associated with higher levels of support seeking in both online and face-to-face environments (Davison et al. 2000, p. 214)—the very circumstances that typify the experience of infertility.

The exponential growth of single-function OSGs has generated a burgeoning field of research, especially in health psychology and related clinical/health sciences. There are far fewer studies in sociology, where interest in computer-mediated communication focuses more broadly on the uses of social media (e.g. Chambers 2006); research methods for digital data (e.g. Waller et al. 2015); self-identity, everyday life and digital practices (e.g. Lupton 2015, 2016); and the maintenance of transnational relationships (e.g. Wilding 2006). In the health sciences, attention has concentrated on the key social and structural characteristics of online support seeking: the asynchronous nature of communication and absence of geographic/temporal barriers, the chance to remain "invisible" and anonymous and the text-based nature of communication (e.g. Barak et al. 2008; Tanis 2007). A key observation frequently made in this literature is that

OSGs attract particularly high levels of self-disclosure (Rheingold 1993; Parks and Floyd 1996; Wallace 1999), far beyond that evidenced in face-to-face groups—and that this is a consequence of the distinctive dimensions of computer-mediated communication.

Our study seeks to fill a gap in the sociological literature by examining the Stronger Together OSG as a narrative environment (Gubrium 2005). Specifically, we focus on the women's accounts of their selfhood and emotions, and their portrayal of the support, conflicts and tension they experienced in their relationships with spouses, parents, siblings and friends in the context of their struggles with infertility. In the chapters that follow, we examine how these various dimensions of the infertility experience are constructed in the online space. How do the women seek support? How do they offer support to one another? How do they construct their identities and how are intimacies produced in the online space? Self and other, identity, meaning making, emotion management, and the intersection of the women's accounts with broader cultural narratives of the self and infertility comprise the micro-sociological lens we adopt in this study. Through analysing excerpts from online journals and posts on the Stronger Together site, we offer a close-up view of women's identities, emotions and support seeking, as they navigate the "roller-coaster" world of infertility. Our micro-sociological work builds on, and advances, extant studies of OSGs in health psychology and the clinical/health sciences literature. This literature provided an important foundation to our study, laying out the key characteristics and effects of health-related OSGs, which we summarise below.

Inspired by Everett Hughes (1984; cited in Gubrium 2005, p. 526), we argue that the social setting of an OSG can be understood as a "going concern": a communicative space that involves "the work of maintaining particular ways of framing and doing matters of relevance to the participants". Participants of Stronger Together were encouraged to emplot their experiences in very particular ways, "positive thinking" being one of the dominant frames in circulation. In Chaps. 3, 4, 5 and 6, we examine the way in which their stories were produced and distributed in the online space. We consider how these stories relate to the various social environments the women inhabit and traverse, in an effort to understand what they "do with words" (Gubrium 2005, p. 525). And we ponder the social consequences of their stories, asking "what is at stake" in their "everyday contexts of storytelling" (Gubrium 2005, p. 525).

The Birth of Support Groups

The phenomenon of the "support group", as we know it today, emerged in the mid-twentieth century through the establishment of Alcoholics Anonymous' 12-step programme in the US, and the subsequent development of other 12-step programmes. "Narcotics Anonymous", "Gamblers Anonymous" and "Overeaters Anonymous" are perhaps the best known of these later iterations. According to Barak et al. (2008, p. 1868), the 12-step model demonstrated that:

> [G]roup support was essential in helping members recover from a distressful situation and obtain some emotional relief. These groups based themselves on the simple premise that people who share similar difficulties, misery, pain, disease, condition, or distress may both understand one another better than those who do not and offer mutual and pragmatic support.

Historically, it could also be argued that support groups had their roots in such fraternal organisations as The Freemasons (Barak et al. 2008, p. 1868), early trade unions and mutual aid organisations. Whereas these associations were involved primarily in practical or material assistance, the fundamental distinguishing feature of contemporary support groups is the provision of peer-to-peer emotional and informational support (Tanis 2007). By way of illustration, Malik and Coulson (2010), in an analysis of the content of 3500 messages posted to a UK-based infertility OSG, reported the most frequently used self-help mechanisms as "support or empathy" (45.5%), "sharing of personal experiences" (45.4%) and "provision of information and advice" (15.9%).

Yet, the increasing popularity of OSGs since their emergence late last century must be seen in the broader context of the rise of therapy culture and several other significant, interrelated social, economic and political changes. This chapter opens with an overview of these contextual factors. Next, in discussing the insights provided by the literature on OSGs from health psychology and clinical/health sciences, we touch on key debates in this field of research and pay particular attention to the self-empowering effects of participating in OSGs—a significant theme in the journals and posts we examined for this project. We then turn to an overview of the key characteristics and effects of OSG participation, utilising related insights from our participants. Finally, we discuss the significance of social support for people's health and wellbeing, an area of research that is important in understanding the rise of online support groups.

Therapy Culture and the "Emotionalisation" of Society

Led by developments in clinical and applied psychology, especially in the fields of education and work and in counselling more generally, the growth of therapy culture has significantly shaped the way people make sense of themselves and their personal difficulties (Brownlie 2014, p. 12; Illouz 1997, 2008; Silva 2013). As Katie Wright (2008) argued, a shift has taken place across the second half of the twentieth century, in particular, from reticence and self-reliance as the culturally dominant approach to dealing with personal distress to an emphasis on emotional expressiveness and help seeking. The ascendancy of psychology as a discursive regime, and the popularisation of psychological knowledge through "self-help" literature and other mass media, has generated a new language of selfhood that calls attention to emotional injuries and vulnerabilities, personal needs and individual wellbeing (Furedi 2004a, 2004b; Illouz 2008). With characteristic deftness, renowned novelist Ian McEwan (2007, p. 26) captured this cultural orientation in *On Chesil Beach* from the perspective of early 1960s Britain:

> The language and practice of therapy, the currency of feelings diligently shared, mutually analysed, were not yet in general circulation. While one heard of wealthier people going in for psychoanalysis, it was not yet customary to regard oneself in everyday terms as an enigma, as an exercise in narrative history, or as a problem waiting to be solved.

This "new" therapeutic language of selfhood, which sees the self "as a problem waiting to be solved", has become embedded in everyday social interactions, beyond the purview of clinical experts and professionals.

We see it voiced in magazines, films, reality television, in such "talk shows" as *Oprah* and *Jerry Springer*, in "coming out" stories, and in the ever-growing popularity of biographies, autobiographies and other "confessional modes of expression" (Greco and Stenner 2008, p. 3; Holmes 2016, p. 28; Illouz 2008). In an examination of newspaper representations of major Australian bushfires between 1939 and 2009, Duffy and Yell (2014, p. 106) posited that the use of mobile phones/digital cameras to send messages and images of natural disasters to radio and television stations, even as these events were unfolding, is contributing to "an emphasis on the therapeutic function of the media as a space in which to give expression to traumatic and other difficult feelings". Advances in electronic communications technology and the growth of various social media platforms have coincided with the rise of therapy culture, arguably intensifying its effects (Gibson 2016; Walter 2007).

Yet, it is not only the media that drives our pervasive attention to the self in late western modernity. In recent decades, the realm of the emotional has become increasingly apparent as a frame of reference for understanding and evaluating situations and for shaping our actions in all sectors of social life, prompting some critics to claim that an "emotionalisation" of society has occurred (Greco and Stenner 2008, pp. 3, 5; see Brownlie 2014, p. 12). In the criminal justice system, practices of restorative justice provide opportunities for victims of crime to confront their perpetrators over the impacts of their crimes, thereby delivering a form of emotional retribution. In the education sector, "child-centred" teaching practices emphasise open dialogue and emotional engagement between student and teacher, and a shift away from didactic approaches. Even in the political arena, as Greco and Stenner (2008, p. 4) observe, "people expect to see, and experience, emotional engagement. Prominent politicians now routinely sport caring and smiling facial expressions, where once it was compulsory to look stern and disciplined."

Of particular relevance to the present study, the philosophies and practices of "individualised" or "person-centred care" encourage health professionals to focus on patients' needs and choices and their emotional wellbeing (Yeatman 2009). The growth of consumer health movements, along with the weakening of hierarchical relationships between service users and health professionals and the questioning of their expert knowledge (Beck 1992; Giddens 1991) form part of a broader set of influences that constitute the ongoing democratisation and individualisation of society (Beck and Beck-Gernsheim 2002; Coontz 2004; May 2013, pp. 22–38; Wright 2008). So, too, these developments are tied to the growth of consumer culture and consumerism, which, as Joan Busfield (2011, p. 4) points out, has "enhanced the public's desire for its needs and wants to be satisfied … expectations are typically higher, and demands greater and more likely to be given voice". To complete the picture of our socio-historical terrain, we may add the far-reaching effects of second wave feminism, civil rights movements and the contemporary focus on human rights, all of which have helped to produce and reinforce the significance of emotions and emotional wellbeing in every sector of life. Thus the very broad influences, enumerated in this section, provide a frame through which to contextualise and explain the proliferation of OSGs as venues for emotional help seeking, information and support in late modernity. We might also surmise that the intimate exchanges that characterise OSG participation both shape and are shaped by the language of therapy, now "in general circulation" (McEwan 2007, p. 26).

Key Debates in the Research Literature on Online Support Groups

Early research into single-function OSGs focused on the benefits and disadvantages of using this (relatively) "new" form of support. Key benefits were usually defined in terms of the unique features of computer-mediated communication: the asynchronous and text-based nature of communication; the absence of geographic and transportation barriers; opportunities to expand one's social network; and, the relative anonymity or "invisibility" afforded by the online environment (Tanis 2007; see Barak et al. 2008; Suler 2004).

The potential for "uninhibited, aggressive, and socially inappropriate remarks or *flaming*" (Fingeld 2000, p. 250; italics included) and for inaccuracies in health information were seen as the main disadvantages of participating in an OSG (Hinton et al. 2010; Mo and Coulson 2014).

Nonetheless, given the number and range of individuals on most sites, it was assumed that others would rectify the posting of incorrect and unreliable information in a timely manner (Bartlett and Coulson 2011, p. 113; Chung 2013, p. 1408; Fingeld 2000, p. 250). Moreover, as Fingeld (2000, p. 250) noted, individuals who participate in health related OSGs are "for the most part … highly invested in constructive communication".

Additionally, Malik and Coulson (2010), in their content analysis of 3500 messages posted to a UK-based infertility OSG, found very few posts (0.3%) contained negative statements. The majority of these "negative" statements revealed feelings of pain and sadness when learning of the treatment successes of other participants (Malik and Coulson 2010, p. 317). In an earlier study, based on a questionnaire with open-ended questions, the authors (Malik and Coulson 2008a, p. 110) noted that some participants felt that occasional misinterpretations of the content of postings "were exacerbated by the stressful nature of fertility treatment, which made many members highly sensitive to the remarks of others". They concluded that their content analysis upheld the findings of previous studies, which show that "online support groups provide many of the helping techniques found in face-to-face support groups and very few instances of negative or disinhibited communication", and that their study indicated "the key functions of this online support group were to exchange support and empathy and provide a forum for individuals to share their personal experiences related to infertility" (Malik and Coulson 2010, p. 318).

Another concern voiced in the literature is that of the "therapeutic efficacy" of OSGs (Fingeld 2000, p. 253; see Malik and Coulson 2010, p. 318) compared with "traditional" face-to-face "therapy" groups (White and Dorman 2001, p. 693). However, the question of which form of support is more effective seems to us beside the point. The OSG and the face-to-face therapy group are qualitatively different in process and function, and cater to different needs. Barak et al. (2008, pp. 1869–70) have identified five key differences. First, there is no compulsory targeted or planned treatment programme in support groups; second, the main purpose of a support group is to "offer *relief and improved feelings* rather than therapeutic change" (Barak et al. 2008, p. 1868; italics included); third, support groups usually function without leaders or administrators whereas therapy groups are run by qualified professionals; fourth, a support group is open to anyone who wishes to join or simply "lurk" on the site, whereas therapy groups are generally restricted to those who "sign-up" to them; and fifth, therapy groups are usually time-limited whereas support groups are not (Barak et al. 2008, pp. 1869–70). The literature review conducted by Barak et al. (2008) is especially helpful in making sense of concerns about the therapeutic efficacy of OSGs. They reported "little or no specific outcomes" for individuals participating in OSGs, although there is much evidence for such "nonspecific personal impacts" as the fostering of emotional wellbeing, self-confidence, sense of control, and social interaction, all of which are "highly important psychological factors" (Barak et al. 2008, p. 1867; see Bartlett and Coulson 2011, pp. 113–4). As Barak et al. (2008, p. 1869; italics added) explained:

> Support groups, including their online version, are not a substitute for the treatment of any kind of distress. A common mistake … holds that a good support group might replace therapy. The argument made here, however, is that participation in a support group—perhaps even more so in an online support group—might in many cases *provide added value to standard therapy, counselling, or professional care … as this means of emotional support has the great potential to contribute to participants' sense of personal empowerment.* As such, online support groups might be considered a possible supplement to more traditional professional treatment; their contribution lies more in affecting people's general well-being than causing therapeutic change.

Some critics have cautioned against the possibility that involvement in OSGs may lead participants to distance themselves from in-person contact (Barak et al. 2008, p. 1867; Chung 2013). However, these concerns seem unfounded according to the literature. Common sense might suggest that individuals who receive inadequate support from their offline relationships are more likely to seek it from online sources, compared with those who receive adequate levels of support from family and friends. However, the opposite seems to be true. According to Shaw et al. (2006), cited in Chung (2013, p. 1410), individuals with greater support from family and friends reported more frequent use of OSGs than those with lower levels of offline support. Could it be that people with higher levels of offline support are more active and engaged in their support seeking and support utilisation processes; that is, they are more active in offline *and* online spaces? As Chung (2013, p. 1410) surmised: "Online and offline worlds are psychologically connected and felt and experienced as continuous spaces … so offline social relationships are expected to influence the way one communicates on the Internet." While our research project was not designed to test this argument, it is an interesting one nonetheless. We know that many of the women who posted to Stronger Together complained about the lack of support and understanding they received from "real life" relationships and, in some cases, as we show in the following chapters, non-infertility sufferers were seen as "the enemy". It was certainly the case that many of the women sought support from a range of medical and allied health professionals, and from family and friends, while also seeking support from the OSG. However, we cannot know whether the women who were active on the Stronger Together site were more active in seeking offline support than IF sufferers who were not involved in an OSG.

Furthermore, the women in our study used the OSG as a supplement to formal support and treatment services, not as a replacement for these more conventional services. Many commented that their sense of isolation had been reduced as a result of participating in the OSG, and that they felt supported, heard and understood. These generalised (rather than specific) effects, which were very important to the women, can be understood in terms of the experience of personal empowerment, a concept we unpack below.

The Empowering Effects of OSG Participation

Drawing on the work of Staples (1990), Barak et al. (2008, p. 1869) argued that "empowerment refers to experiencing personal growth as a result of developing skills and abilities along with a more positive self-definition", and involves both "perceived capabilities in coping" with a range of difficulties and challenges and "perceived ability" to deal with problems in the future. The term "sense of empowerment", often used in the literature and by lay people, denotes "an *experiential mental state* rather than an objective condition" (Barak et al. 2008, p. 1869; italics and emphasis added). According to Barak et al. (2008, p. 1869) there are three main facets of personal empowerment: self-reliance and reliance on other group members with similar experiences, rather than professionals, which engenders a sense of personal mastery; voluntary participation in the OSG, which creates a sense of self-determination and control; and involvement in helping others and relating first hand to their experiences, which facilitates experiences of social engagement.

Another way of conceptualising personal empowerment is that it centres on self-care and self-reliance, and dealing with emotional difficulties *outside* professional and health service involvement. As we will see from later discussion in this chapter, the key features of computer-mediated communication, often designated as "advantages" in the literature, also function as potential generators of personal empowerment for people in distress. Conditions of anonymity, invisibility, and asynchronous and text-based communication foster openness, intimacy and a sense of belonging. Barak et al. (2008, p. 1872) identified five main ways in which personal empowerment is produced in the context of OSGs. First, the process of writing itself "enables emotional outlet and a sense of cognitive order" (Barak et al. 2008, p. 1872). Referring to a study of participants' story-telling in a Scandinavian breast cancer OSG, Hoybye et al. (2005) found that:

[B]y sharing personal stories with others in the group, [participants] were actively portraying their life stories and identities. The shift from being acted upon to being active in inter-subjective storytelling and taking charge of themselves through the written word results—as these researchers reported—in an elevated sense of control and empowerment. (Barak et al. 2008, p. 1873)

Second, the process of sharing painful emotions, which often brings emotional relief and a sense of unburdening, creates "feelings of belongingness and togetherness [that] are crucial and significant, and contribute to personal empowerment" (Barak et al. 2008, p. 1874). Third, personal empowerment can flow from receiving and providing information;

factual information and suggestions about coping strategies provide encouragement and hope, and are often more "easily accepted, than receiving the information from a professional" (Barak et al. 2008, p. 1875). Fourth, the forming of relationships in the OSG environment provides a sense of belonging, affiliation, and social cohesion—a safe place for people who feel "isolated and different" (Barak et al. 2008, p. 1875). This sense of empowerment may also have positive effects on participants' formal offline relationships, as Chung (2013, pp. 1412–13) suggested:

> Through the use of information on the Internet, including OSGs, patients can strengthen their ability to question the quality of care received from healthcare professionals … Empirical evidence suggests that the Internet serves as an additional and complementary resource for health information but does not displace the role of healthcare professionals … [and] patients' use of the Internet … reflects their desire to participate in healthcare.

Fifth, conditions of heightened self-confidence and reassurance generated through OSG participation are likely to enable better decision-making and "behavioural transformation":

> Discussions among group members challenged participants to rethink and revaluate their prior decisions, attitudes, and courses of action in regard to coping with their emotional, social, and practical difficulties. The process of rethinking and revaluating provided greater understanding of relevant issues and more confidence in taking action. (Barak et al. 2008, p. 1876)

We can see this transformative dimension of empowerment exemplified in Simone's response to Erin's post on the (public) discussion board of Stronger Together. In great exasperation, Erin, who wanted a baby "so badly", had posted that she did not know "how much more" waiting she could tolerate in her quest to fall pregnant. She loathed "having to try so hard", and had been attempting to convince herself that "surely" it would happen with time, and she would bypass "all the hoops that other women have to jump through" (i.e. IVF, the ups and downs of continual monitoring, and the endless waiting for test results). She had begun to realise, however, that she was probably "no different" from other women struggling with infertility and would have to "suck it up" and get on with the necessary tests and interventions. Concluding her post with "I just hate it!" imparted a plea for help: How can I deal with the myriad stresses of medical procedures and the uncertainties of success or failure? Through identifying with Erin's experiences in opening her response ("I felt the same way for over a year"), Simone normalised Erin's emotions, while communicating understanding and compassion. She then suggested that "jumping" through all "those hoops" was but a small price to pay, should a pregnancy eventuate; thus by rethinking and altering her "perspective" in this way, Erin could help herself adjust to the realities of the situation. This form of support, frequently provided in the OSG, illustrates the potentially transformative, and empowering, aspects of participation engendered through reassurance from a fellow sufferer (Barak et al. 2008, p. 1876). In micro-sociological terms, this exchange constitutes a cognitive strategy of interpersonal emotion management (Hochschild 1979) (see Chap. 5).

Malik and Coulson (2008a), in a questionnaire-based study, referred to earlier, explored the online experiences of women and men who accessed online infertility support groups in the UK. The sample was made up of 95 individuals, 94% of whom were women. Questions focused on participants' motivations for accessing online support and their experiences of support seeking (i.e. perceived advantages and disadvantages of online support participation, and the effects of this support on coping with infertility and in negotiating their marital relationships). Participants identified a range of significant benefits from their online participation that appeared to facilitate their coping responses to the "psychosocial challenges" they faced in diagnosis and treatment of infertility; in other words, they viewed their participation as empowering. Four of the five key themes that emerged from the authors' inductive thematic analysis of the data clearly reflected the experience of personal empowerment. The first, depicted as "unique features of online social support" included the site's 24-hour availability, the asynchronous nature of online communication and the anonymity involved in the exchanges, enabling them to "speak" of painful and negative emotions without embarrassment, and have "breathing space" before posting responses (Malik and Coulson 2008a, pp. 107–8). The second theme concerned "improved relationships" with their partners; opportunities to discuss a range of anxieties and stresses with one another seemed to take some of the strain off their marital relationships. In this regard, the site offered "a valuable source of emotional support and positive encouragement"; as a consequence some women reported "becoming more sympathetic to their partners' emotions and coping strategies surrounding infertility" (Malik and Coulson 2008a, p. 108). The third theme, designated as "reduced sense of isolation", focused on the significance of communicating with others who had first hand experiences of infertility; this reduced participants' feelings of guilt and abnormality and helped to normalise their emotional responses (Malik and Coulson 2008a, pp. 108–9). The fourth theme, "information and empowerment", referred to situations of increased awareness and knowledge of treatment options which followed in the wake of interactions in the OSG, enabling participants to assume a more active role in decision-making concerning their treatments (Malik and Coulson 2008a, p. 109).

As noted above, Barak et al. (2008, p. 1879) argued that the objective of OSGs—and support groups in general—"should be seen in terms of affording general emotional relief and an elevated sense of control—two essential components of personal empowerment … That is, when evaluating the impact of a support group on participants in terms of general, nonspecific effects, findings show a quite different picture from conclusions that address therapeutic effectiveness". Furthermore, drawing on a study by Barak and Dolev-Cohen (2006) of an OSG for suicidal adolescents, Barak et al. (2008) emphasised that participation in an OSG does not provide a "sufficient condition" for "emotional relief" or "an elevated sense of control". In this unobtrusive analysis of the postings of group members over a period of three months, the authors found that "on average" participants did not experience a sense of emotional relief. However, the more active participants, "in terms of responding to others and being responded to" obtained emotional relief compared with the more passive participants (Barak et al. 2008, p. 1879). This finding suggests that "active participation" is important in generating "greater personal empowerment" (Barak et al. 2008, p. 1879). Perhaps this is not surprising: the process of *involvement* itself, whether through seeking or providing support, helps produce a sense of unburdening, social engagement and belonging, aspects of online exchanges that are inherently comforting and empowering.

Characteristics and Benefits of Online Support Groups

OSGs are structured in two main ways. Health professionals and health-care services moderate some groups, delivering expert advice, assessment and individually focused programs. In Fingeld's (2000, p. 243) words, these groups provide a "comprehensive" version of online interactive support. Membership tends to be limited to individuals who "sign-up" or are referred to the group by a professional to complete a specific pro-gramme. The other, more commonplace, form that pertains to our study is an "open" online space where group membership is voluntary and people "come and go" as they wish, the aim being to "provide a forum in which individuals with similar concerns can support each other" (Fingeld 2000, p. 243).

A range of internet-based technologies have been used in setting up OSGs. The most basic form in the early history of OSGs was a list of email addresses through which members could communicate with one another, often with "listserver" software used to automate and streamline this process (Tanis 2007, p. 140). "Chat rooms" are also used, but a dis-cussion forum ("bulletin board") is by far the most common application (Barak et al. 2008, p. 1868; Tanis 2007, p. 140). Members can post mes-sages to the "board" for others to read and comment on, and can initiate new "threads" whenever they wish. In addition to a forum, some OSGs invite participants to create their own personal journals to which other members may respond as they would to postings on a general forum. The OSG on which this book is based offers a general forum, as well as space for personal journals and several other options for supportive interac-tions. Because discussion forums are generally open to all visitors, close relatives and care-givers may gain information and insights into the particular illness or form of distress which, in turn, can assist them in understanding and supporting their loved one (Tanis 2007, p. 140).

Asynchronous Communication

Because of the asynchronous nature of computer-mediated communication, participants may post comments and journal entries, respond to questions, and initiate new threads, 24-hours per day. Most significantly, participants have the capacity to control how and when they post to the site. They can take their time to prepare and edit posts, to consider very carefully the content they are releasing into cyberspace (White and Dorman 2001, p. 694). Specifically, support providers can take time in constructing their support messages to reflect on what is being written; to ensure that their messages are sensitive and clear, given the text-based mode of communication and the high levels of distress often presented by people seeking support (Chung 2013, p. 1409). Because participants engage and interact in the online environment from the comfort of their own homes and other settings, any geographic, temporal or transportation barriers that may hinder access to formal face-to-face support are removed (Tanis 2007; White and Dorman 2001, p. 694; Chung 2013). In the absence of time-space barriers, OSGs also enable people to expand and diversify their social support networks (Tanis 2007), circumstances especially beneficial for people who are homebound or live in geographically isolated areas.

A cursory scan of the discussion board of the OSG on which this study is based shows that newcomers to the site received supportive replies and welcome messages very quickly, often within ten minutes of posting. The speedy responses to Bronwyn's post are a case in point. She made her initial post to the general discussion forum at 10.25 am. Introducing herself, she explained that she was in her late 30s and had been "TTC for 2 years". Bronwyn prefaced her story by saying she needed "some support and discussion" from women who shared her struggles. Recently, she had undergone surgery to remove fibroids, after which she felt very hopeful of falling pregnant. Unfortunately, according to her doctor, she had very few "good eggs" left and he advised a course of fertility drugs and hormone injections. Not keen to go down this route, she wanted to try "the natural way"—but "holding onto hope" was proving very difficult since she had already experienced several pregnancy-like episodes (e.g. "sore boobs"), all eventuating in "crushing" defeat when her period appeared. Bronwyn's cycles were in disarray; sometimes early, sometimes late, so she couldn't be certain when, or if, ovulation had occurred. Currently her body was telling her she might be pregnant, so Bronwyn was trying to resist convincing herself of this joyful possibility, in an effort to prevent another plunge into misery. Her post exemplified the very high levels of self-disclosure often expressed in OSG interactions, with the audience taken into the intimacies and intricacies of her bodily reactions and thoughts as she struggled to cope with the ups and downs of infertility. Like many other women on the site, she sought advice on how to manage this roller-coaster ride: the challenge of maintaining hope amid the frequently shifting ground between excitement and despair. Admitting to the occasional "complete break-down" and feeling sorry for herself, she noted for the most part that she was "positive". Thus she embraced the dominant narrative of "staying positive" (see Chap. 4), while demonstrating her efforts to take responsibility for her own wellbeing (Crawshaw 2012, p. 201).

Bronwyn received her first response from Francine at 10.31am; she empathised with Bronwyn's "struggles", urging her to "stay positive", and hoping that her body's symptoms were actual "pregnancy signs". She sent "lots of luck" and affirmed that Bronwyn had "come to the right place for support". Francine's response was brief. She did not offer specific strategies through which to maintain hope beyond her entreaty to "stay positive". What is important is that her message was "selectively attuned" (Chung 2013, p. 1409) to the emotions Bronwyn had expressed. In this way, Francine recognised her "struggle" and offered hope and understanding. The second response came from Victoria at 10.40 am. She strongly identified with Bronwyn's plight, revealing that she and her partner had also been "trying" for two years. Like Bronwyn, she had undergone surgery and wanted to utilise "natural" interventions, noting her use of Mayan abdominal massages and a plan to investigate essential oils. Both her opening statement ("Hugs to you") and closing remark ("Best of luck") were conversational and intimate in tone, evoking the comfort and familiarity of close friendship. Both Francine and Victoria's exchanges generated a strong sense of empathic support, as evidenced in Bronwyn's reply at 10:57 am: "Thanks guys! :) I swear I feel better already."

The more emotive posts—those in which the initiator wanted "to vent" or was desperately seeking emotional advice and support—tended to elicit speedier responses and a greater number of them, compared with posts inquiring about specific medical treatments. For example, one post titled "DHEA or Progesterone Causing Cystic Acne?" had received no replies after a week, whereas posts titled "Why are expected negatives so disappointing?" and "Coping with my emotions" received several responses within an hour of posting.

Invisibility and Anonymity

The "invisible" presence of the self in computer-mediated communication means that any anxieties about one's appearance and voice are removed from the encounter. These conditions can themselves be disinhibiting, giving people "the courage to say things they otherwise might not" (Barak et al. 2008 p. 1871). The absence of such nonverbal cues as frowning or dismissive looks, which could inhibit people in face-to-face encounters, may also add to the "powerful online disinhibition effect" (Barak et al. 2008, p. 1867), identified by numerous researchers (e.g. Singleton et al. 2016; Suler 2004; Tanis 2007). Most notably, individuals with stigmatising or embarrassing problems, who might otherwise be marginalised from support seeking, can seek and receive support without needing to be troubled by these problems (White and Dorman 2001, p. 694).

Similarly, the opportunity to remain anonymous also encourages discussion of discomfiting, sensitive or otherwise "taboo" topics (Collin et al. 2011; Malik and Coulson 2008a; Suler 2004; Tanis 2007). Malik and Coulson (2008a, p. 111), in their questionnaire-based study of the experiences of individuals accessing infertility OSGs in the UK, reported that "the anonymous nature of an online forum was thought by many to be a key advantage when discussing painful and negative emotions", a finding also made in studies of other health-related OSGs (e.g. Barak et al. 2008; Fingeld 2000; Suler 2004). In the online setting, people tend to feel less vulnerable, less concerned with "losing face" (Chung 2013, p. 1409). One need not feel ashamed or that one's privacy will be violated (refer to Chap. 3). Furthermore, in some face-to-face settings the act of receiving support can make the support seeker feel helpless and beholden to the person providing the support, whereas this dynamic is ostensibly weakened or even absent in the online context of anonymity.

The benefits of anonymity in the Stronger Together online environment were championed by Kate in a post she made to the general forum. Here she revealed her efforts to prepare both mentally and physically for an upcoming IVF cycle. Like many other participants on the site, she described the alternative therapies she had been utilising (acupuncture and vitamins). Foremost, however, she focused on the need to control her high stress levels and myriad anxieties concerning unforeseen medical complications, in an effort to give herself the best possible chance of success. In terms of working on herself, she articulated the goal of forgiving herself "for being stressed", so as to prevent herself from "stressing about being stressed". In concluding her post, she expressed gratitude for the opportunity to "put myself out like this", noting that in other settings she would shy away from disclosing her innermost thoughts for fear of being criticised or feeling "crazy". She felt accepted, understood and at ease in this online environment. Her post also illustrated the intricacies of the self-governance of one's wellbeing through the "work" of self-monitoring and self-improvement (Crawshaw 2012; Petersen 1996). (See Chap. 4.)

As McKenna and Bargh (2000, p. 62) noted: "Under the protective cloak of anonymity users can express the way they truly feel and think", generating possibilities for self-disclosure. Considering this phenomenon at a more abstract level, Joinson (2001) surmised that anonymity in online settings reduces "public self-awareness" and feelings of accountability, thus making self-disclosure more likely. Moreover, the sensitive and very personal nature of the topics discussed in single-function (health-related) OSGs tend to generate and intensify practices of self-disclosure. The emotional freedom to reveal one's inner thoughts and feelings is presumably facilitated, at least in part, by the private, familiar and safe settings from which posts are made and otherwise potentially awkward questions are asked. Yet a further factor that fosters individuals' emotional freedom to self-disclose is the neutralising of status (Barak et al. 2008,

p. 1872) produced by the online environment: "Respect comes from one's skill in communicating, the quality of one's ideas, and one's integrity as a person. Everyone, regardless of status, wealth, race, or gender, starts off on a level playing field" (Barak et al. 2008, p. 1872).

Thus one's invisibility and anonymity in the setting of OSG interactions help to produce high levels of interpersonal intimacy and empathy, and focused social support and bonding. As we will show throughout the following chapters, supportive messages online were "often selectively attuned to the situations and emotions of support recipients" (Chung 2013, p. 1409). Drawing on Collins' (2004) work on interaction ritual chains, we posit that the "emotional energy" generated in online interactions "provides a sense of group solidarity … that can create recurring participation" (Jasper 2014, p. 209). That is, we can trace the "'emotional entrainment' of successful interactions" (Jasper 2014, p. 209) through the carefully focused attention from support provider to support recipient. Because support messages are exchanged in largely text-based form in OSGs, the "supportive intention tends to be clearly presented" (Chung 2013, p. 1409), as the following exchange demonstrates. Siri, the newcomer initiating this particular thread, sought advice from others as to how she might keep her hopes up and stay positive in the face of despair. Siri stated that she was "losing hope": she felt it ebbing away from her, and each day she seemed to have "less and less". With her thoughts constantly focused on "having a baby", the sight of pregnant woman, including many of friends, made her "cry inside"; and, she no longer knew what to say to people who asked when she and her DH would be starting a family. In a seemingly beseeching manner, she asked how other women on the site kept "sane" and maintained their hope.

Debbie, the first respondent, assured Siri she had "come to the right place", where she could "vent" and share her fears with others who would understand her experiences. She then revealed how she herself had dealt with the ongoing sense of loss and failing hopes, while being careful to acknowledge that she, too, "bounces" around with highs and lows, and fluctuating emotional states that are difficult to control. Not wanting to "sugar coat" the roller-coaster reality of the infertility experience, Debbie admitted that she, too, had very "little hope" at times. As she explained, however, she cultivated hope from several sources: from reading "success stories" on the site, from her friends, and "most of all" from her spiritual/ religious faith.

Tatum, the second respondent, echoed Debbie's advice to Siri, while also responding to Siri's particular concerns. She revealed that she, too, suffered the "ups and downs" of infertility, and felt demoralised in encountering pregnant women "all around" her, especially those who had fallen pregnant after only a couple of months of "trying". Through addressing both Siri and Debbie in her conversational moves, the emotional entrainment of a successful interaction was achieved (Jasper 2014, p. 209). Tatum noted how the site had helped her enormously and added, as Debbie "mentioned", that Siri would find many others going through "the same experiences". Developing her response a little further, and contributing to "a sense of group solidarity" (Jasper 2014, p. 209), she emphasised that people who had never experienced infertility "don't understand what we're dealing with" and many of their attempts at support—including advice to "just relax" and "take a vacation"—did not help. Building on Debbie's point, she concluded her post by affirming that she, too, enjoyed reading "success stories" on the site because they offered hope that "all the hard work" she was putting in with her DH may "possibly" be rewarded. Connecting with Debbie's point also reinforced a collective sense of belonging to a community of similar others. In reply, Siri thanked them for their advice, revealing that her interaction with them had already reduced her sense of isolation and she felt "lucky" to have communicated with women confronting similar dilemmas and emotions. The emotional energy generated by Siri's cry for help produced a sense of "group solidarity" with the two respondents reflecting back her emotions and revealing the depth of their own very similar struggles. Through the conversational moves in this exchange, Debbie and Tatum "worked" to encourage Siri to become more hopeful—to provide her with tools to rethink and adjust to her situation. Their supportive moves signify an interactional achievement—a form of interpersonal collaborative emotion management (Hochschild 1979, 1983) or "hope work" (Gengler 2015).

Researchers have put forward two main theories as to why high levels of intimacy and self-disclosure develop in online support groups

(Chung 2013, p. 1409). One holds that anonymity gives rise to greater openness that generates intimate relationships. The other, rooted in social comparison theory (Festinger 1954), concerns the "strong feelings of commonality" individuals experience from participating in an online community; that is, a sense of group identity tends to develop in the context of connecting through similar, distressing experiences (Chung 2013, p. 1409). Applying Festinger's social comparison theory to interactions in OSGs, we can argue that people need to compare themselves with similar others, especially under situations of stress and uncertainty:

> Social comparison is part and parcel of the process of social validation in which people use relevant groups they are part of to establish meaning, values and identity ... Importantly, social validation is best achieved when people can compare themselves with others that are relatively similar to them (and whose experiences are therefore diagnostic to the self). The availability of similar others makes online support groups a good stage for social comparison purposes. (Tanis 2007, pp. 145–6)

As we show in this chapter and throughout the book, social comparison also enables people to learn how to understand and cope with their difficulties.

Text-Based Communication

Almost the entire content of interactions in the OSG environment are text-based, granted that participants also have at their disposal a (growing) range of emoticons to help communicate their intended meanings. Seminal work by Pennebaker and colleagues (Davison et al. 2000; Pennebaker 1997; Pennebaker and Seagal 1999) demonstrated that the act of writing about one's personal and emotional difficulties can be therapeutic in itself, largely because of the cognitive and emotional changes involved in producing the account. In revealing traumatic experiences and painful emotions to others, one must construct a comprehensible account of these experiences (Davis 2000; Pennebaker 1997). Through the process of sequencing, explaining and providing insights into these very particular circumstances, the individual creates for herself a deeper, clearer, more organised and fundamentally "storied" understanding of the meaning of her experiences. In addition, as Barak et al. (2008, p. 1873) explain, "[t]hrough writing, the writer expresses thoughts and emotions that may not have been and are difficult to be exposed in other environments."

The act of exposing one's innermost feelings and thoughts may ameliorate the person's sense of loneliness, their isolation and lived distress, leading to an experience of emotional relief and catharsis (Finn 1995; Miller and Gergen 1998; Symth et al. 1999). In a similar vein, sociologist Joseph Davis (2000, pp. 36–7) identified three main functions involved in storying the self. First, the meaning of particular experiences and events is clarified. Secondly, the process involves a therapeutic function by facilitating a "working through" of stressful events, engendering positive adaptation and coping; these experiences are often rendered more bearable and therefore may help to strengthen the person's self-image (see Chap. 4 for several in-depth examples of "working through"). Thirdly, storying the self is fundamental to a person's identity, and accounts of self are organised through various modes of emplotment (Frank 1995, 2010; Ricoeur 1991). Narratives of positive thinking and (associated) self-empowerment, and individual responsibility, comprised two of the dominant plots utilised in the posts and journals we examined for this project.

The Significance of Social Support

It has long been established in the social science literature that social support contributes significantly to a person's physical and mental wellbeing (Brown and Harris 1978; Cobb 1976; Cohen and Wills 1985). According to Tanis (2007, p. 139), social support refers to "a whole range of ways in which people can tacitly or explicitly help one another to improve the quality of their lives … [it] is found to be beneficial for reducing stress, decreasing feelings of loneliness and isolation, getting hold of knowledge and information and learning strategies to cope with the situation people are facing". As discussed above, social support can also enhance

individuals' self-care and self-esteem, and foster their sense of empowerment. More recently, medical science has demonstrated through numerous studies that social support and social connection are linked with an
improved immune system and longevity (e.g. Cacioppo and Patrick
2008). Social support may benefit individuals directly by providing a
sense of belonging and connection to others, and fostering self-care, for
example, and indirectly through affording a buffering effect against the
deleterious consequences of stress and uncertainty (Kawachi and Berkman
2001; Turner and Brown 2012).

Social support tends to be conceptualised in the literature in three
qualitatively different forms: "instrumental", "informational" and "emotional" forms of assistance (Tanis 2007, p. 140; see House and Kahn
1985). Instrumental assistance includes such practical tasks as helping
with shopping, housework and transportation to appointments, and is
therefore less relevant to the practices of OSGs than the two other forms.
Informational assistance involves exchanging knowledge about medical
and non-medical treatments, test results, and legal and financial issues.
The women in our study frequently sought and provided this form of
assistance to one another, as illustrated in the following excerpt from
Patricia's online journal:

> I will be sure to ask my RE when I see her on Monday but I wanted to
> know if anyone has been told to avoid exercising when doing stims and
> after transfer?
>   I am so tired of the extra 15 pounds I have put on the past 6 months
> during all of this IF stuff! HATE the gym, but DO belong and haven't gone
> in almost a year … I have to do SOMETHING! I am so uncomfortable in
> my own skin! I have typically been a fairly in shape woman. Never really
> concerned with more than losing 5–10 pounds (can't we all). But now I
> could stand to lose a good 20 lbs and get rid of all the fat dimples on my
> legs and butt and the extra muffin top!

Romana responded, noting that she, too, had put on 15 pounds. Even
while eating in a very "healthy" way, "the pounds keep coming", so she
reasoned that it had to be caused by the "IVF drugs". As a consequence,
her RE "now" recommended gentle exercise after transfer, albeit with the

proviso not to engage in "any movement that could shake a ponytail". Given the different opinions of reproductive endocrinologists, Ramona encouraged Patricia to check with her own specialist for advice on exercise following a transfer.

Not surprisingly, emotional assistance has been identified as the most common form of support in OSGs (Tanis 2007, p. 141; see Malik and Coulson 2010), as noted above—a finding also borne out through the women's journal excerpts and general forum posts we examined in our study. This affective form of support involves communicating understanding and compassion. Most importantly, "empathy plays a vital role" (Tanis 2007, p. 141) through the provider of support showing that she feels the feelings of the recipient, offering encouragement for further self-expression, and suggesting specific coping strategies and ways of reframing particular dilemmas. Emotional support is especially beneficial in situations people are unable to change (e.g. Wright 2000), a common characteristic of the situations experienced by infertility sufferers.

In the following exchange initiated by June, a newcomer to the site, the provider of support responded empathically, reflecting back to her the feelings she had expressed and offering several practical suggestions and ways of re-imagining her situation. In opening her post, June explained that she was 25 years old and had been "trying" for a baby for three years. The Stronger Together site had been recommended by a work colleague. June described feeling "sad" every time her period arrived and admitted not knowing "where to go to get tested" for infertility. In particular, she was distressed by her mother "guilting" her for not providing a grandchild. June surmised that her mother must not know "how much it hurts me" to see other people's babies and to hear her frequent reminders concerning grandchildren. She also assumed that her mother probably did not realise she could be infertile. June admitted being at a loss over what to do and "just" wanted to get these worries "off my chest" and "see" what others thought.

Olivia responded very compassionately, exclaiming deep sorrow on learning of June's emotional suffering, and wished she "never" had to be "among us" at such a young age. She strenuously advised her to make an appointment with a "good fertility expert", through the help of her local doctor. There was a chance, she cautioned, that the "obstacle" preventing conception may be curable, especially if treated in its early stages, as in the case of PCOS (Polycystic Ovarian Syndrome). She urged her not to "waste" her time on the site, but to see a specialist in an effort to gain an accurate diagnosis of the problem and possibly resolve it.

Olivia then turned to the matter of June's mother, and encouraged her to try to see the situation from her mother's perspective. She suggested that she try not to "get insulted" by her attitude; to recognise that her mother probably did not know how stressful June's experience of "unknowing" could be. She pressed June to initiate an open dialogue with her mother: a "heart-to-heart talk" to tell her how "difficult" things were for her and affirm that she definitely wanted to provide grandchildren, but needed her support and understanding to "move on more confidently" in an attempt to resolve the issue. This exchange exemplified how empathy and advice were frequently offered in the online space: Olivia empathised with June's situation, encouraged her to rethink her relationship with her mother by considering her mother's perspective (and thus enlarging her view of the situation beyond her immediate feelings), and provided advice on how to take action to foster her own self-care. This example illustrates the potentially transformative and empowering aspects of OSG participation (Barak et al. 2008, p. 1876).

Some of the women in our study used the Stronger Together site to seek emotional assistance for perceived difficulties in their relationships with their husbands, particularly over matters of support and in sharing responsibility for planning and financing treatments (Steuber and Solomon 2008) (see Chap. 6). In a journal entry, Caroline expressed deep concern that she and her husband were "not on the same page" in saving for IVF treatments:

> This is really petty but I must vent. DH bought me an ipad for my bday. This is after he got me an iphone for x-mas and I asked him to return it. Here I sit, struggling to save for IVF treatments and he keeps buying me expensive gifts that I don't need. I haven't bought myself anything new for probably a year. My priority is to save for IVF. His priorities are different. We are not rich. DH busts his ass working side jobs for extra cash. He has not once asked or offered to help save for IVF stuff. We keep our money separate. It just makes me sad that we are so far apart on this. I feel guilty even writing this. He's trying to be nice. I should be grateful.

Three fellow participants responded to Caroline's dilemma, offering understanding and compassion and a means of rethinking the situation. Merran revealed that she and her husband had experienced a similar predicament. She offered Caroline an alternative frame for re-imagining the dynamics in her relationship with DH: "guys just have different mindsets". From this perspective, Caroline's DH is not selfish, even though he has not asked about or offered to save for IVF. It is because he is a man that he sees and responds differently to the situation. The person is not at fault; it is his gender that has produced him as "different" from her.

In providing advice to Caroline, both Georgie and Leanne built on Merran's lay theory of fundamental gender differences. Georgie reinforced this view, explaining that men "deal with IF differently" and "cope differently" and he simply "can't help" his views because he is "a guy". She encouraged Caroline to go beyond an immediate surface-level reading of DH's behaviour to appreciate the apparent care and concern underlying his efforts, surmising that he was probably "just feeling like he was doing something nice" to "make you happy". Taking the cue from Georgie, Leanne argued that men often assume that gift giving will make "everybody feel better" and they fail to "think deeply enough" to comprehend that such expensive gifts are upsetting when the money could have been put aside to finance the IVF procedures. She then offered a practical strategy, aimed at defusing the hostility Caroline was feeling towards her DH: that she tell him "how sexy he'd be" if he deposited the money into her IVF account, rather than purchasing "flashy gifts". Echoing Georgie's view, she speculated that his gifts were very likely motivated by a desire to alleviate her sadness but, like other men, was "out of touch" with "exactly" what to do in the given situation. Leanne offered an analytical frame through which Caroline might re-imagine her situation. The seeming impasse between them was not simply a matter of the DH's personal failings, but part of a bigger picture of gendered social conditioning. The three respondents built progressively on one another's posts, each attuned to Caroline's emotions and, together, providing an alternative lens through which to view DH's behaviour in a positive light, thus constituting a form of collaborative emotion management (Harris 2015, p. 50). Caroline thanked the three "ladies", affirming that their input was "really … helpful. DH is just trying to cheer me up for sure". Again, this example demonstrates the potentially transformative and empowering aspects of OSG participation (Barak et al. 2008, p. 1876), and shows that emotions are "profoundly interpersonally influenced … shaped by and jointly constructed with others" (Gengler 2015, p. 612).

In a recent interview-based study of infertile couples, Hinton et al. (2010) found that the provision of emotional support was seen as the most significant function of OSGs, lending strong support to earlier findings in the literature and to the findings of our study. Hinton et al. (2010, p. 437) explored the question of how and why couples were using the Internet for support, in order to identify the positive and negative effects of "niche support online". The 38 women and men who participated in their study were asked to describe their support needs and "where" and "how" they attempted to meet them. Hinton et al. (2010, pp. 436–7; italics added) noted that:

> The Internet offers anonymity, emotional support, normalisation and reassurance … from others who are going through treatments at the same time and in similar circumstances … While interviewees often talked about unpleasant physical aspects of treatment *it is the emotional and social consequences of their infertility that stand out in their descriptions.*

Some of the participants interviewed by Hinton et al. (2010, p. 439) explained that their involvement in an OSG helped to bolster their offline relationships with spouses and friends by providing another "outlet", thereby reducing the need to discuss and "obsess" over their problems with significant others. In a similar vein, the exchanges between Caroline, who wanted to "vent" about her seemingly unsupportive husband, and the three Stronger Together respondents (Merran, Georgie and Leanne), illustrate how the cultivation of "weak" ties in the online environment may help to preserve participants' "strong" ties in offline contexts. The internet enables "new communities of support that supplement the real world" and provides access to other people's perspectives and experiences (Hinton et al. 2010, p. 440). The sharing of personal experiences online both fosters and is fostered by the broader emotionalisation of society (Greco and Stenner 2008), which inspires the forging of individualised, "niche" identities—a theme that is taken up in Chaps. 4 and 5.

Conclusion

We opened this chapter by contextualising the phenomenon of online support groups in relation to the rise of therapy culture and such related social processes as the growth of consumer health movements, and the democratisation and individualisation of society. Then, drawing on recent studies of OSG participation in the field of health psychology and clinical/health sciences, we argued that the fundamental distinguishing feature of these online groups is the provision of peer-to-peer emotional and informational support (Tanis 2007). Emotional support is particularly meaningful for people experiencing conditions that are felt to be embarrassing or stigmatising, or cannot be changed—characteristics that frequently define the experience of infertility. Several examples of support seeking and support provision were presented to show the micro-social details of *how* empathy is offered and received in the online environment of Stronger Together. Support provision in the form of specific coping strategies, including the reframing of individual circumstances, can be conceptualised as interpersonal emotion management (Harris 2015, p. 50; Hochschild 1979). This micro-sociological lens is especially constructive for analysing the "moves" made by our participants in the context of their online interactions. In this chapter, we also set out our particular contribution to the sociological field of infertility studies. By examining Stronger Together as a very particular narrative environment, we aim to show how particular stories are encouraged, and produced and circulated in the online space. In Chap. 3, we focus on the online environment as a community of support; Chap. 4 analyses the women's construction of their selves and identities; Chap. 5 focuses on their relationships with significant others (family members, friends and work colleagues); and Chap. 6 explores the women's relationships with their spousal partners.

References

Barak, A., & Dolev-Cohen, M. (2006). Does Activity Level in Online Support Groups for Distressed Adolescents Determine Emotional Relief. *Counselling and Psychotherapy Research, 6*(3), 186–190.

Barak, A., Boniel-Nissim, M., & Suler, J. (2008). Fostering Empowerment in Online Support Groups. *Computers in Human Behavior, 24*(5), 1867–1883.

Bartlett, Y. K., & Coulson, N. S. (2011). An Investigation into the Empowerment Effects of Using Online Support Groups and How This Affects Health Professional/Patient Communication. *Patient Education and Counseling, 83*(1), 113–119.

Beck, U. (1992). *Risk Society: Towards a New Modernity*. Newbury Park: Sage.

Beck, U., & Beck-Gernsheim, E. (2002). *Individualization: Institutionalized Individualism and Its Social and Political Consequences*. London; Thousand Oaks, CA: Sage.

Brown, G. W., & Harris, T. (1978). *Social Origins of Depression: A Study of Psychiatric Disorders in Women*. Tavistock: London.

Brownlie, J. (2014). *Ordinary Relationships: A Sociological Study of Emotions, Reflexivity and Culture*. London: Palgrave Macmillan.

Busfield, J. (2011). *Mental Illness*. Cambridge: Polity Press.

Cacioppo, J. T., & Patrick, W. (2008). *Loneliness: Human Nature and the Need for Social Connection*. New York: Norton.

Chambers, D. (2006). *New Social Ties: Contemporary Connections in a Fragmented Society*. Houndmills; New York: Palgrave Macmillan.

Chung, J. E. (2013). Social Interaction in Online Support Groups: Preference for Online Social Interaction Over Offline Social Interaction. *Computers in Human Behavior, 29*(4), 1408–1414.

Cobb, S. (1976). Social Support as a Moderator of Life Stress. *Psychosomatic Medicine, 38*(5), 300–314.

Cohen, S., & Wills, T. A. (1985). Stress, Social Support and the Buffering Hypothesis. *Psychological Bulletin, 98*(2), 310–357.

Collin, P., Metcalf, A., Stephens-Reicher, J., et al. (2011). ReachOut.com: The Role of an Online Service for Promoting Help Seeking in Young People. *Advances in Mental Health, 10*(1), 39–51.

Collins, R. (2004). *Interaction Ritual Chains*. Princeton, NJ: Princeton University Press.

Coontz, S. (2004). The World Historical Transformation of Marriage. *Journal of Marriage and Family, 66*(4), 974–979.

Crawshaw, P. (2012). Governing at a Distance: Social Marketing and the Bio(Politics) of Responsibility. *Social Science & Medicine, 75*, 200–2007.

Davis, J. (2000). Accounts of False Memory Syndrome: Parents, "Retractors", and the Role of Institutions in Account Making. *Qualitative Sociology, 23*(1), 29–56.

Davison, K. P., Pennebaker, J. W., & Dickerson, S. S. (2000). Who Talks? The Social Psychology of Illness Support Groups. *American Psychologist, 55*(2), 205–217.

Duffy, M., & Yell, S. (2014). Mediated Public Emotion: Collective Grief and Australian Natural Disasters. In D. Lemmings & A. Brooks (Eds.), *Emotions and Social Change* (pp. 99–116). Oxford: Routledge.

Festinger, L. A. (1954). A Theory of Social Comparison Processes. *Human Relations, 7*(2), 117–140.

Fingeld, D. L. (2000). Therapeutic Groups Online: The Good, the Bad, and the Unknown. *Issues in Mental Health Nursing, 21*(3), 241–255.

Finn, J. (1995). Computer-Based Self-Help Groups: A New Resource to Supplement Support Groups. *Social Work with Groups, 18*(1), 109–117.

Frank, A. (1995). *The Wounded Storyteller: Body, Illness & Ethics*. Chicago: University of Chicago Press.

Frank, A. (2010). *Letting Stories Breathe: A Socio-Narratology*. Chicago: University of Chicago Press.

Furedi, F. (2004a). *The Therapy Culture: Cultivating Vulnerability in an Uncertain Age*. London; New York: Routledge.

Furedi, F. (2004b). Reflections on the Medicalisation of Social Experience. *British Journal of Guidance & Counselling, 32*(3), 413–415.

Gengler, A. (2015). "He's Doing Fine": Hope Work and Emotional Threat Management Among Families of Seriously Ill Children. *Symbolic Interaction, 38*(4), 611–630.

Gibson, M. (2016). Youtube and Bereavement Vlogging: Emotional Exchange Between Strangers. *Journal of Sociology, 52*(4), 631–645.

Giddens, A. (1991). *Modernity and Self-Identity: Self and Society in the Late Modern Age*. Cambridge: Polity.

Greco, M., & Stenner, P. (2008). *Emotions: A Social Science Reader*. London: Routledge.

Gubrium, J. F. (2005). Introduction: Narrative Environments and Social Problems. *Social Problems, 52*(4), 525–528.

Harris, S. R. (2015). *An Invitation to the Sociology of Emotions*. Abingdon; Oxford: Taylor & Francis.

Hinton, L., Kurinczuk, J. J., & Ziebland, S. (2010). Infertility; Isolation and the Internet: A Qualitative Interview Study. *Patient Education and Counseling, 81*(3), 436–441.

Hochschild, A. R. (1979). Emotion Work, Feeling Rules, and Social Structure. *American Journal of Sociology, 85*(3), 551–575.

Hochschild, A. R. (1983). *The Managed Heart: Commercialization of Human Feeling*. Berkeley, CA: University of California Press.

Holmes, K. (2016). Talking About Mental Illness: Life Histories and Mental Health in Modern Australia. *Australian Historical Studies, 47*(1), 25–40.

House, J. S., & Kahn, R. L. (1985). Measures and Concepts of Social Support. In S. Cohen & S. L. Syme (Eds.), *Social Support and Health* (pp. 83–108). Orlando, FL: Academic Press.

Hoybye, M. T., Johansen, C., & Tjornhoj-Thomsen, T. (2005). Online Interaction: Effects of Storytelling in an Internet Breast Cancer Support Group. *Psycho-Oncology, 14*(3), 211–220.

Hughes, E. C. (1984). *The Sociological Eye*. New Brunswick, NJ: Transaction Books.

Illouz, E. (1997). Who Will Care for the Caretaker's Daughter? Toward a Sociology of Happiness in the Era of Reflexive Modernity. *Theory, Culture & Society, 14*(4), 31–66.

Illouz, E. (2008). *Saving the Modern Soul: Therapy, Emotions, and the Culture of Self-Help*. Berkeley, CA: University of California Press.

Jasper, J. M. (2014). Constructing Indignation: Anger Dynamics in Protest Movements. *Emotion Review, 6*(3), 208–213.

Joinson, A. N. (2001). Self-Disclosure in Computer-Mediated Communication: The Role of Self-Awareness and Visual Anonymity. *European Journal of Social Psychology, 31*(2), 177–192.

Kawachi, I., & Berkman, L. F. (2001). Social Ties and Mental Health. *Journal of Urban Health, 78*(3), 458–467.

Lupton, D. (2015). *Digital Sociology*. Abingdon: Routledge.

Lupton, D. (2016). *The Quantified Self: A Sociology of Self-Tracking*. Cambridge: Polity.

Malik, S. H., & Coulson, N. S. (2008a). Computer-Mediated Infertility Support Groups: An Exploratory Study of Online Experiences. *Patient Education and Counseling, 73*(1), 105–113.

Malik, S. H., & Coulson, N. S. (2008b). The Male Experience of Infertility: A Thematic Analysis of an Online Infertility Support Group Bulletin Board. *Journal of Reproductive and infant psychology, 26*(1), 18–30.

Malik, S. H., & Coulson, N. S. (2010). Coping with Infertility Online: An Examination of Self-Help Mechanisms in an Online Infertility Support Group. *Patient Education and Counseling, 81*(2), 315–318.

May, V. (2013). *Connecting Self to Society: Belonging in a Changing World*. Basingstoke: Palgrave Macmillan.

McEwan, I. (2007). *On Chesil Beach*. New York: Doubleday.

McKenna, K. Y. A., & Bargh, J. A. (2000). Plan 9 from Cyberspace: The Implications of the Internet for Personality and Social Psychology. *Personality and Social Psychology Review, 4*(1), 57–75.

Miller, J. K., & Gergen, K. J. (1998). Life on the Line: The Therapeutic Potentials of Computer-Mediated Conversation. *Journal of Marital and Family Therapy, 24*(2), 189–202.

Mo, P. K. H., & Coulson, N. S. (2014). Are Online Support Groups Always Beneficial? A Qualitative Exploration of the Empowering and Disempowering Processes of Participation Within HIV/AIDS-Related Online Support Groups. *International Journal of Nursing Studies, 51*(7), 983–993.

Parks, M. R., & Floyd, K. (1996). Making Friends in Cyberspace. *Journal of Communication, 46*(1), 80–97.

Pennebaker, J. W. (1997). Writing About Emotional Experiences as a Therapeutic Process. *Psychological Science, 8*(3), 162–166.

Pennebaker, J. W., & Seagal, J. D. (1999). Forming a Story: The Health Benefits of Narrative. *Journal of Clinical Psychology, 55*(10), 1243–1254.

Petersen, A. (1996). Risk and the Regulated Self: The Discourse of Health Promotion as Politics of Uncertainty. *Australia and New Zealand Journal of Sociology, 31*(1), 44–57.

Rheingold, H. (1993). *The Virtual Community: Homesteading on the Electronic Frontier*. Reading, MA: Addison-Wesley.

Ricoeur, P. (1991). Life in Quest of Narrative (trans. D. Wood). In D. Wood (Ed.), *On Paul Ricoeur: Narrative and Interpretation* (pp. 20–33). London: Routledge.

Shaw, B. R., Hawkins, R., Arora, N., McTavish, F., Pingree, S., & Gustafson, D. H. (2006). An Exploratory Study of Predictors of Participation in a Computer Support Group for Women with Breast Cancer. *CIN: Computers, Informatics, Nursing, 24*(1), 18–27.

Silva, J. (2013). *Coming Up Short: Working-Class Adulthood in an Age of Uncertainty*. New York: Oxford University Press.

Singleton, A., Abeles, P., & Smith, I. C. (2016). Online Social Networking and Psychological Experiences: The Perceptions of Young People with Mental Health Difficulties. *Computers in Human Behavior, 61*(August), 394–403.

Slauson-Blevins, K. S., McQuillan, J., & Greil, A. L. (2013). Online and In-Person Health-Seeking for Infertility. *Social Science & Medicine, 99*(December), 110–115.

Staples, L. H. (1990). Powerful Ideas About Empowerment. *Administration in Social Work, 4*(2), 29–42.

Steuber, K. R., & Solomon, D. H. (2008). Relational Uncertainty, Partner Interference, and Infertility: A Qualitative Study of Discourse within Online Forums. *Journal of Social and Personal Relationships, 25*(5), 831–855.

Suler, J. (2004). The Online Disinhibition Effect. *CyberPsychology & Behavior, 7*(3), 321–326.

Symth, J. M., Stone, A. A., Hurewitz, A., & Kaell, A. (1999). Effects of Writing About Stressful Experiences on Symptom Reduction in Patients with Asthma or Rheumatoid Arthritis: A Randomized Trial. *Journal of the American Medical Association, 281*(14), 1304–1309.

Tanis, M. (2007). Online Social Support Groups. In A. N. Joinson, K. Y. A. McKenna, T. Postmes, & U.-D. Reips (Eds.), *The Oxford Handbook of Internet Psychology* (pp. 139–153). Oxford: Oxford University Press.

Turner, R. J., & Brown, R. L. (2012). Social Support and Mental Health. In T. L. Scheid & T. N. Brown (Eds.), *A Handbook for the Study of Mental Health: Social Contexts, Theories and Systems* (pp. 200–212). Cambridge: Cambridge University Press.

Wallace, P. (1999). *The Psychology of the Internet*. Cambridge: Cambridge University Press.

Waller, V., Farquharson, K., & Dempsey, D. (2015). *Qualitative Social Research: Contemporary Methods for the Digital Age*. Los Angeles: Sage Publications.

Walter, T. (2007). Modern Grief, Postmodern Grief. *International Review of Sociology, 17*(1), 123–134.

White, M., & Dorman, S. M. (2001). Receiving Social Support Online: Implications for Health Education. *Health Education Research, 16*(6), 693–707.

Wilding, R. (2006). Virtual Intimacies? Families Communicating across Transnational Contexts. *Global Networks: A Journal of Transnational Affairs, 6*(2), 125–142.

Wright, K. (2000). Computer-Mediated Social Support, Older Adults and Coping. *Journal of Communication, 50*(3), 100–118.

Wright, K. (2008). Theorizing Therapeutic Culture: Past Influences, Future Directions. *Journal of Sociology, 44*(4), 321–336.

Yeatman, A. (2009). *Individualisation and the Delivery of Welfare Services*. New York: Palgrave Macmillan.

3

Finding Support in the Online World

Paulina Billett

"To end this journal, I just want to say THANK YOU to all you ladies who have been here for me, supporting me and giving me advice. I really do appreciate all of it, and all of you!" Joan

When most people think of online relationships, their mind usually summons the spectre of countless "cat-fish" and internet "predator" stories which abound in the tabloid media. These cautionary tales would lead us to believe that the online environment produces relationships that are damaging and often misleading due to our inability to clearly ascertain who we are dealing with in a physical sense. It is this sense of the unknown, the anonymity of others, which has cemented popular opinion of online relationships as somehow inferior, less intimate and more fleeting than offline relationships (Hart 2015). Yet, our research shows that this is not necessarily the case. Instead, our research posits, as others have before us

P. Billett (✉)
La Trobe University, Melbourne, Australia
e-mail: p.billett@latorbe.edu.au

© The Author(s) 2019
P. Billett, A.-M. Sawyer, *Infertility and Intimacy in an Online Community*,
Palgrave Macmillan Studies in Family and Intimate Life,
https://doi.org/10.1057/978-1-137-44981-8_3

63

(e.g. see Chambers 2013) that the relationships formed between members of online communities, such as Stronger Together, are highly supportive, extremely intimate and as enduring as those formed offline. Furthermore, these relationships can have far reaching positive impacts, both emotionally and psychologically for those seeking support. Findings such as these have challenged how we conceptualise "intimacy" and "relationships" (Chambers 2013) and suggest that we may need to move towards new understandings of these terms which emphasise the value individuals derive from their online relationships.

The wide array of social practices which are described as "intimate" in the online setting demand a significant shift in how we think of intimacy between individuals. Before the challenges of the online world, intimacy was conceptualised only in terms of face-to-face contexts. Intimate relationships were seen to exist only in the realm of the personal/domestic, present between family and friends, and entailing some manner of exclusivity, romantic and/or sexual attachment (Chambers 2013). The rise of the online environment and its capacity to "blend" the boundaries of the public/private, and familiarity/indifference has shifted the landscape in seismic proportions. As such, we claim that for many individuals, such as the women of Stronger Together, the online environment represents new ground where support is gained and relationships are formed, constituting the first node of the relationship triangle.

In this chapter, we continue the conversation which we begun in Chap. 2 on the role OSGs play in the mental and physical wellbeing of their members by exploring this first node. We begin with a general description of the changes to intimacy in the twenty-first century and examine how these shifts have helped to create spaces in which individuals, who may not find support in offline relationships, can find fertile ground for companionship and support in the online world.

Changes to Intimacy in the Twenty-First Century

It can be argued that changes to our understanding of intimacy and intimate relationships in the twenty-first century encompass only the latter parts of a much wider set of social changes which began in the mid- to late twentieth century. This shift, which included the rise of second wave feminism, changes to family structure and increase in the visibility of gay and lesbian couples, saw the loosening of traditional bonds and the rise of "elective bonds" such as "friends as family" becoming increasingly common. This, it is suggested, has led to a detraditionalisation of intimacy and a reconfiguration of its "performance" (Gross 2005).

According to Giddens (1992), the democratisation of the "interpersonal domain" in late modernity has led to a shift in intimacy from the traditional romanticised forms to a confluent model which emphasises choice and compatibility with individuals, and engagement in a "reflexive" project of the self in which one chooses the makeup of their intimate relationships. The "pure relationship", a term Giddens uses to describe "a situation where a relationship is entered into for its own sake", is largely based on benefits derived by each individual and is "continued only in so far as it is thought by both parties to deliver enough satisfactions for each to stay within it" (Giddens 1992, p. 57). This type of relationship is now dominating the landscape of intimacy in the twenty-first century. Most importantly, intimate relationships, rather than being seen in terms of traditional familial ties and obligation, are instead judged by a "culture of self-fulfilment, supported by therapeutic ideologies" (Chambers 2013, p. 44).

However, not everyone sees the deconstruction of traditional intimacy as a successful, or desirable shift. Those such as Bauman (2003) and Beck and Beck-Gernsheim (1995) fear that this democratisation has in fact led to self-interest and a weakening of social bonds. In his book *Liquid Love* (Bauman 2003) Bauman suggests that traditional bonds are loosening their holds, allowing relationships to become ambivalent as well as impermanent, leaving individuals feeling highly vulnerable, all the while fearing the restriction relationships bring. Bauman (2003) writes:

Our contemporaries, despairing at being abandoned to their own wits and feeling easily disposable, yearning for the security of togetherness and for a helping hand to count on in a moment of trouble, and so desperate to "relate"; yet wary of the state of "being related" and particularly of being related "for good", not to mention forever—since they fear that such a state may bring burdens and cause strains they neither feel able nor are willing to bear, and so may severely limit the freedom they need.

Similarly, Beck and Beck-Gernsheim in their book, *The Normal Chaos of Love*, suggest that individualism, together with the romanticising ideal of absolute love, has aided in the breakdown of traditional paradigms of permanent relationships, which has instead been replaced by "partner of the moment" relationships, giving way to a multiplicity of family configurations. In *Distant Love*, they set out what they call "the global chaos of love"; the creation of "every conceivable kind of relationship at a distance" created by the rise of globalised mobilisation and more particularly by the globalised mediums of virtual communication (Beck and Beck-Gernsheim 1995, p. x) and the difficulties individuals face in maintaining these relationships.

While the bleak pictures painted by Bauman and Beck and Beck-Gernsheim of modern romantic love are compelling, they do not account for the potential gratification these looser relationships may bring, or the ways in which these ties may in fact be helping to redefine community. In our analysis of the stories provided by the women of Stronger Together, we align ourselves more fully with Giddens, in suggesting that the relationships formed in the OSG, which are ultimately based on choice and companionship, rather than loosening or breaking down social bonds, help to create a new type of community based on friendships and serving an essential purpose in the lives of the women by generating much needed emotional support. Thus, these ties, rather than generating anxiety, can work as a "shield", helping the women to cope with the uncertainty produced by their diagnosis—as attested to by the plethora of posts and journal entries that seek advice, comfort and support from others.

OSGs, such as Stronger Together, have been found to be valuable sources of emotional support as well as fostering self-empowerment (Barak et al. 2008). van Uden-Kraan et al. (2008) suggest that participating in OSGs, as either a poster or a "lurker", has many positive effects, and allows participants to feel "better informed; more confident with their physician, their treatment, and their social environment; improved acceptance of the disease; increased optimism and control; and enhanced self-esteem and social well-being."

Empowerment is a multidimensional concept encompassing, social, spiritual, political, economic and psychological dimensions and to bring about desired results (Barak et al. 2008) (See Chap. 2 for a discussion of self-empowerment in OSGs). For the individual, empowerment may mean the ability to make more informed decisions about treatment, to access support and understanding in times of need, and procure advice on personal matters. According to Dickerson (1998) self-help groups are one of the most effective ways of promoting individual empowerment.

Reaching out to a support group often occurs due to a desire to belong to an entity which is composed of individuals who share similar issues and who may provide understanding which is lacking in offline interaction. As discussed in later chapters, many of the women who frequented Stronger Together encountered or perceived negative attitudes towards their infertility journey, either from society or from significant others, resulting in the view that the offline world can be a hostile environment from which they need to retreat (see especially Chaps. 4, 5 and 6). The online support group provides these women with a place in which to "gather" and discuss issues they feel are likely to be misunderstood by others, especially topics relating to "negative feelings" such as jealousy and resentment. It is thus unsurprising that many posts and journal entries we encountered tended to reflect four distinct, yet at times connected, topics: information seeking, venting, grief and joy. Of these, it was the discussions of more negative manifestations—anxiety about treatment and the grief of infertility (often seen as unacceptable in the "offline" world), which the women suggest have brought the most comfort.

Information Seeking

The expression of negative emotions online has been found to improve wellbeing and quality of life for support group participants (Lieberman and Goldstein 2006). The anxiety created by treatment and the possibility of failure was by far the most frequently displayed negative emotion among the women in both their posts and journals. The loss of control over one's body was for many the hardest aspect of infertility and fertility treatment. The intense medicalisation of their body was accompanied by a demystification of the reproduction process while X-rays, ultrasounds, and blood tests, rather than producing answers, mechanised the process of reproduction, leading them to see their bodies as little more than faulty machines which fail to do what "normal" bodies do. Thus, many women stopped seeing their bodies as part of themselves, and instead began to discuss them as somehow removed and in terms of conditions and ensuing interventions (e.g. blocked tubes, inhospitable cervix, low motility, female factor, male factor, unexplained infertility to name but a few).

Their desire to feel in control and to understand their condition drove the women to become pseudo-experts. It was not unusual for women to write lengthy detailed entries of their treatment cycles, which contained highly specific medical information. For most individuals without a medical degree, these entries would read as excerpts from medical journals. However, for these women, their immersion in medical terminology and test results had become a way of life; an important "lifeline" to make sure they were able to participate in their treatment. As Nadine posted in her journal:

> Well the Embryo Transfer went well this morning. I had 3 very high grade 2 morula's [sic] and two other 8 cell embabies that are also grade 2. DH, RE, the embryologist and I debated back and forth as to how many to transfer [sic] back and finally decided on 4 (the 3 Morulas and one of the 8 cell embryos. I feel really good about that decision.

Often journal entries like these elicited responses from a number of online friends who offered support and reassurance by posting encouragements or offering their own experiences with medication or treatment. This helped to relieve anxiety and assured the women that all was well. However, the benefits of sharing this medical knowledge goes further than the recipient as, according to Barak et al. (Barak et al. 2008), conveying information to others is also an important part of the self-empowerment process because it transforms the individual from information seeker to an information provider, who possesses vital and valuable experience and information and is able to provide support to others. As such, by sharing information, the women were able to regain control in a highly uncontrollable situation and demonstrate to themselves as well as others their level of knowledge and authenticity.

For some, posting notes on treatment to the site or in their journal was also a coping mechanism used when they felt that treatment was not progressing as it should. The relationships which the women built were often used as platforms for assurance. Seeking information from others on the site allowed those undergoing treatment to feel empowered and to challenge the medical establishment. For example, Joan, after becoming frustrated with her doctor at being "left to my own devices as regards my medical cycles", seeks the help of others on Stronger Together in determining what testing and monitoring should be conducted. She states that she has had little to no contact with her RE and no monitoring has been conducted aside from blood test. After giving an account of her past medical testing, which showed ovulation, she then compared this to her previous RE by stating:

> I've had several ultrasounds done to check for cysts and the state of my uterus; I've had blood work to check my hormone levels; and I've had an HSG done.

She then asks:

> Is there anything you ladies can suggest to me that I should 'demand' my RE or even GP test me for?

What is more, we often saw responses encouraging the questioning of medical expertise, and frequently women were given suggestions of further questions or procedures, which they should "ask" their doctors to answer or undertake. As such, the participation in an OSG such as Stronger Together has created a new type of patient, one who is well informed and no longer willing to be a "passenger" in her treatment. As Mary discussed in her journal:

> … The numbers got scribbled down and she was out the room, at no change in 5 days I asked why, then she was called back in and said—ok we will change your medicine to Menapor—(just like that) … if I had not asked what my numbers were would have she bothered?

Journals or posts discussing poor "bed side manner" were responded to with a high degree of sympathy for the member's situation and anger towards treating physicians and their staff. We often witnessed calls from other members for the women to change doctors and seek better care, or to directly question their doctors about their treatment. Many women felt that the focus placed on their bodies by the ART process dehumanised their struggle and it was up to them to remind practitioners of their needs. The new paradigm created by the rise of OSGs has meant that fertility clinics and their staff need to deal with increasingly savvy patients who will not easily tolerate what they feel to be a disengaged or substandard approach to their treatment. This no-nonsense attitude has meant that many fertility clinics are being challenged to create new practices of care, which emphasise the patient's needs and their individual journey within treatment. This sharing of information as a form of support is not surprising, as research has shown that a sense of self-empowerment is achieved when knowledge is acquired outside authority filtering agents, such as medical experts (Barak et al. 2008).

Venting

"Venting", as the women of Stronger Together call this, entailed the sharing of negative emotions such as anger, resentment and jealousy. Venting was the second most common form of posting after seeking medical information on Stronger Together for many women. Venting provided a rare source of release, comfort and understanding, what many women stated to be the place they could go to really be themselves. In these types of entries, women spoke of their struggles with the feelings of inadequacy, their resentment of pregnant women, their frustration with partners and family (see Chaps. 4, 5 and 6). For them, this was a place to which they could come and express those feelings which they felt would not be understood by "others". An example of this can be seen in Lilli's journal entry where she writes about her frustration at finding out that one of her nephew's girlfriend is pregnant again:

> I just need to vent! last night we had dinner with my MIN [mother in law] and BIL [brother in law] … it was all very lovely until my mother in law turns around and says to me, did you know that Cameron and Holy are expecting? I nearly fell over backwards! my mouth literally was hanging

open for around 5 seconds and I think all I said was oh nooooo! This is my 24-year-old unemployed, mooching off his father nephew and his 20-year-old, mother of one (whose father only god knows who it is) at 16, unemployed, can't even look after her first child girlfriend! What are these two going to do with another baby! My nephew was doing well until he met this woman, he had a great job as an IT professional for a large company, earning great money and looking forward to travelling and then she came along … it's been about a year and he quit his job (because he had to stay home to take care of her and her baby when she doesn't work???!!!) is living with her and her kid at my BIL's house without paying for a single thing (my BIL can't stand this girl but felt he couldn't kick out his son) and now they have a baby on the way!!!! … It's so unfair, what kind of life will they be giving this child! how can they fall pregnant just like that! … I know this sounds selfish, but now I will have to cope with seeing all this mess unfold while I am longing so desperately to have a baby, knowing that my child would have had a great life with DH and I, that she would have been loved so much, we would have done everything in our power to make her life happy … and while I know it is far away still I am already dreading this year's Christmas, once again without a baby (let's not kid ourselves, its been 5 almost 6 long years 1 IVF, a miscarriage and 3 FETS. Chances of me being pregnant even by Christmas by natural means are nil) and then there will be them, this pair of losers with their little miracle on the way … God forgive me but today I am the bitterest person on the face of this earth …

Posts are also used to vent in a similar fashion. In one post Madeleine describes her jealousy and anger at a friend's pregnancy after just two months of trying. In her post she states that she "can't help it but I'm pissed" and she is "having a hard time being happy for her" as she is "the only one of my friends that is having a problem getting pregnant and it's so easy for everyone else". At the end of her posts she asks for perspective, by writing,

What do I do? How can I shake this anger? I'm having a really hard time this weekend.

Several women join the conversation, assuring her that she is being reasonable and as one reply states "that it is ok to be angry and selfish right now. You don't need to deal with pregnant women if you don't want to".

By far, the members most often vented about the insensitivity of others and, as discussed in Chap. 5, the most common perpetrators were family and friends. Thus, for many women relationships in the offline world become rather precarious, particularly when friends and family members become pregnant or had young children of their own.

The strong emotions aroused by the infertility journey led to those venting often using strong language as a display of raw feelings and emotions which they believed to be "unacceptable" in the offline world. Similarly, grief announcements were used by members as a way in which to display emotions perceived to be unacceptable and to relieve the sadness which is often present and needs to be negotiated during the rollercoaster ride of treatment and failure.

Treatment failure often left the women feeling overwhelmed, and the lack of support from family, partners or the wider society drove many women to the point of exasperation. Posts due to miscarriages were particularly poignant and the women's grief and bitterness was palpable. Many expressed the incomprehensibleness of the situation and cursed at the cruelty of the experience. Many perceived their miscarriage as a double failure, not only was their body faulty and unable to reproduce "naturally" but now they also had failed in "keeping baby safe". These posts almost always received many replies, with women on the site expressing sympathy at the loss. For many of those unfortunate enough to post these heart-wrenching notes, the online world offered further solace, as the replies of other members and messages of concern also meant a validation of their pregnancy and of their loss, something which women who experience miscarriage (particularly at the early stages) often discuss as missing from friends and family responses.

Grief

Grief over failed cycles was also very common. In these posts women expressed their perplexity at the situation and many highlighted their embarrassment at having shared their treatment and hopes with those offline only to have it end in failure. Due to reasons discussed in the following chapters as well as the shame of continued failure, as the length of treatment progressed women increasingly refrained from sharing their treatment with those in the offline world. This meant that for many, Stronger Together became their only source of comfort, support and companionship during their journey and the only outlet for the anxiety which infertility causes.

As a result, the analysis of the women's posts and journals showed them to be the embodiment of an ongoing internal dialogue about the experiences of infertility which could only be shared with trusted others. They were also a way of acknowledging and bringing attention to emotional injuries and vulnerability brought about by the infertility journey. Not surprisingly, the relationships formed in support sites such as Stronger Together are often highly reciprocal and very strong, suggesting a high level of copresence between individuals.

Building Intimacy and Copresence in Stronger Together

Copresence or the perception of mutual entrainment between actors was until recently only understood to encompass physical interactions. However, those such as Campos-Castillo and Hitlin (2013) have argued that the way in which we build and experience copresence and intimacy in our face-to-face relationships is no way different to how this occurs in the virtual world. In fact, it is increasingly argued that physical closeness may not be necessary, but instead, only the perception of "closeness" is required for copresence to exist. In line with this, Campos-Castillo and Hitlin (2013) argue that copresence is not a given, but is subjective in nature, resides in the perception of a connection and is the result of three interlinking components; mutual attention, emotion and behaviour. Mutual attention "refers to a situation in which two actors are reciprocally focused on one another" and this attention in turn enables the establishment of mutual emotion (empathy). Finally, once mutual attention and emotion have been established, actors begin to create automatic or intentional behavioural mimicry, what is referred to as the Chameleon Effect (Campos-Castillo and Hitlin 2013, p. 172) and allows for subjective closeness to be established.

It is not surprising that many of the women who frequented Stronger Together seemed to experience high levels of copresence. After all, the architecture of Stronger Together, coupled with the women's experiences of shared grief, anxiety, hope and joy allowed for the establishment of high levels of mutual attention, emotion and behaviour. For example, the ability to "friend" others, leave messages on member's journals and posts as well as sending virtual "hugs" (which included sentiments such as "there with you", "flowers", "high fives", and "prayers" among others) further helped to create a feeling of shared attention. Further to this, most of our participants where highly active in the community, writing journals entries, and posting or leaving comments and "hugs" several times a week. These messages often contained an element of support for the writer, whether this was in support of their situation, a reassurance and advice or to imply a validation of the writer's position. An example of this can be seen in the following journal entry posted by Lilly after Mother's Day. She writes:

> I survived it … However, I hid away from the entire world for the day … I feel bad that I didn't even see my mother. It is the first Mother's Day we have spent apart, but I really just couldn't get myself together … Also I got a little spotting which means that AF is just around the corner, it was the last thing I needed on Mother's Day and on top of it all, I just comfort ate all afternoon and now I am paying for it. It's just all so wrong … When will there be light at the end of this tunnel!

The replies to her entry, many of them from regular posters, showed high levels of empathy with a number of them acknowledging having done "the same thing", while others professed "I know exactly how you feel". Several posts further sought to validate Lilly's decisions by assuring her that "It's totally ok that you had to hide away today" and "*HUGS* You made it through a really hard day, I'm proud of you. Let's hide from the world if we want and eat junk as much as we feel. We are the only one that knows why". A final post from one friend who often posts on her journal showed the highest possible level of intimacy by stating "love you … plain and simple. I love you dear."

Further to this, we often saw posts and journals which credited the closeness and support received from other Stronger Together members for helping members through difficult times. An example of this can be seen in the following posts and journal entries. At the end of 2012, after a difficult year, which also saw her taking a break from fertility treatment, Carol takes the time to acknowledge the importance of the community in her life and to wish Stronger Together friends a happy Christmas and New Year in her journal. She writes:

> I am so grateful to have options and also grateful for all of you ladies on here who I can share these ups and downs with. Thank you, ladies. I hope you all have a nice holiday. XOXO

Similarly, both Patricia and Elisabeth credit the closeness and support found on the site as integral to their journey. They write:

> It's nice to have this little refuge, where I can come and read success stories to feel inspired, or vent my frustrations. Thank you …! (Patricia)

and

> I joined this site to find support from those that understood how difficult it was to go through this journey … I found that! Thank you everyone for sharing your stories. (Elisabeth)

In each of these journal entries, it is clear that the women feel a unique closeness to one another. For many, the members of Stronger Together are akin to a family group (in fact, members were often referred to by several women as "IF sisters"). For them, there was little need to meet face to face, or to share the same space. What was necessary for closeness and intimacy to exist between support group participants was the shared sense of understanding one another's position and to maintain a sense of connection by the member's participation in forums and journal. Through this, the women forged deep friendships, not at all dissimilar to those one may encounter in the offline world.

However, "sisterly" understanding was not always a given, and the site was not without its problems. It was noted during our time researching that, at least on two occasions, a bitter fight arose between members greatly upsetting for a time the cohesiveness of the group. In the first instance, a member's perceived insensitive comment was highly censored by others. This created tension among a few participants who had "friended" both members and called for calm. Eventually members apologised and the group moved on. However, sometime later, a similar fight erupted between several members. This time, the infighting escalated to the point where one individual was banned by the moderator. Not surprisingly, there was an outcry and many of the women rallied around their friend sending messages to Stronger Together moderators to have the member reinstated. An open thread was created to discuss the situation with no less than three or four pages of posts created over a few days. Many of the women called on others to consider the situation and to email the banned member to "keep her spirits up". Others commented on the importance this individual had on their journey and were angered at the ban and asked for reinstatement of the member. Eventually the banned member returned and a private group was created by those who felt attacked by others. However, within a year or so, all members had re-integrated one again into the general community.

As can be seen, support groups, such as Stronger Together share many of the features of off line relationships, producing high levels of intimacy and copresence without the need for physical shared space. For members, the relationships created and maintained with others are essential and very real. Most importantly, sites such as Stronger Together confirm that "knowing" who we are dealing with in a physical sense is largely unnecessary for copresence and intimacy to exist, as for the majority of women, the anonymity provided by the site was part of its allure.

The Importance of Anonymity in the Online World

Earlier in this chapter we alluded to the important distinction between the offline and online worlds and have suggested that it is the very differences within these realms which make the online world so appealing for those seeking support. In particular, the unique ability of the online environment to obfuscate identity is an essential component in the appeal of online support groups. In fact, anonymity was found in our study to be a vital aspect of the online experience for many women; one that allows the open expression of feelings and attitudes which are often unable to be shared with others in the offline world. What is commonly referred to as the disinhibition effect (Suler 2004; Lapidot-Lefler and Barak 2015).

Much of the discussion surrounding the disinhibition effect has been centred on the rise of e-incivility (e.g. trolling) and its impact on vulnerable individuals. While the debate on e-incivility merits attention, what is often neglected in these deliberations are the benefits which anonymity can have for those who feel their thoughts and feeling may be somehow misunderstood or objected to in the offline world. As we have stated previously, there are some very real therapeutic benefits in the ability to share the anxiety felt when faced by a life altering diagnosis, particularly when those feelings are complicated and seen as objectionable to others. For several women, Stronger Together presented a place where these feelings could be shared without fear of reprisal, in part due to the anonymity afforded by the medium. In fact, our observations of journals and posts demonstrated that women tended to post and journal most often during high periods of stress, and were used as a way of sharing with others their anxieties and fears. In fact, when a word frequency analysis was applied to the women's journals, the words," trying", "positive", "support", "hoping" and "feeling" were among the most often used, suggesting that Stronger Together is a place where hopes and feelings can be shared.

For some such as Joan, the disinhibiting effect allowed her to disclose to her friends on Stronger Together deep feelings of anger arising from interactions with offline family and friends which otherwise would remain "unsaid". In a number of entries, Joan shares profound resentment towards her mother, who she feels does not understand her situation and has failed to support her on her journey. While Joan attends an offline group, it is in the online world where she shaes her feelings and breakes trough with her writting. In her journal she discusses with others how she has come to realise that "I'm still looking for the validation", "I'm still searching for her approval because I feel like I can't do anything right where she's concerned" and that she has come to realise that she is "trying to be the 'perfect daughter' and failing miserably" as she is trying too hard to achieve perfection and that is something she needs to continue working on.

While this realisation was made during her offline support group, it was not until she was within the anonymous environment of Stronger Together that she felt able to share these feelings with others. Moreover, this realisation is not one which she shared with her mother, instead, she continues to write about her volatile mother/daughter relationship in her later journal entries (see Chap. 5).

While the online disinhibition effect is not the only factor that determines how much people open up in the online world, for the women of Stronger Together, it is an important component of their journey. The disinhibiting effect helped the women to gain a sense of empowerment through the expression of suppressed emotions, the improvement of knowledge of treatment options and the increased feeling of "normalcy" over what was often perceived as an otherwise powerless situation. In fact, the ability to "vent" without being fearful of being discovered was an important mechanism utilised by the women at their lowest points, and used by many as a kind of self-therapy, which served to give voice to their feelings and to receive support which validates their position.

However, disinhibition does sometimes come at a price and the thinly veiled anonymity of the online world, could at times be threatened. During our research, it was noted that on at least two occasions, one of the members realised that their online posts were not private, but could be found by anyone simply by "lurking" on the site. This prompted a lengthy discussion by members, with many feeling genuinely panicked by the revelation. The realisation that their words were not just for their online friends but could be directly linked to the rest of their lives was a truly frightening realisation for these women, who felt "ousted" by this new realisation. Lucy opens the thread with the following remark:

> … I only just found out people could [see our post] from all over the web which kinda scared me.

To this, a number of women such as Mimi reply in dismay stating that she "wasn't aware that people from all over the web can read our posts" and those such as Abigail calling on Stronger Together moderators to "please do something about this". Others such as Sharon are more pragmatic stating that Stronger Together "is trying to widen the doors to invite people who need help to find this place easily".

The conversation continues among members with the overwhelming majority preferring to maintain a high level of invisibility from the outside world. This, a number of members acknowledge, would allow them to continue to maintain a high level of disclosure with others without the fear of identification. In fact, the need for anonymity is so great that Penelope, who had only joined a few minutes before decides to leave and find "another site where my privacy won't be violated" rather than chance being "ousted".

Curiously, at least in terms of the members of Stronger Together, disinhibition was achieved through anonymity from offline contact and not between members on Stronger Together. In fact, a number of individuals chose to identify themselves openly in threads which called members to "meet each other". Furthermore, some women also chose to network with one another in the "real world", by either choosing to meet offline or by sharing information such as Facebook profiles during our time of researching. This shift from the totally anonymous realm to the identifiable seemed to happen among members who had frequented Stronger Together for a longer period of time and who had forged deep friendships with others.

Being Friends Off and Online

The rise of the internet in the 1990 heralded a shift in how people could communicate and network. Individuals who may once have felt isolated due to their specific issues where able to find likeminded others in the many groups offered by the online world. Earlier thinking on the online environment suggested that the lack of physical copresence and social context cues meant that online friendships tended to be weaker than their offline counterparts. However, our study as well as many others suggest the opposite, with the friendships forged online becoming an important part of an individual's support network.

As we have already discussed, for many women, their online friendships where outlets for feelings which they did not dare express openly; and the shared experience of hope, loss, heartache meant that their unique connections were credited for helping the members through some of the toughest chapters in their journey. Even after conception and successful delivery, many of the women continued to maintain their friendships on Stronger Together, journaling, lending support to newer members, or sending encouraging messages to those still navigating the labyrinth of fertility treatment. In fact, many of the friendships which were commenced in Stronger Together did not remain within its confines, but instead shifted to more conspicuous arenas, such as face-to-face meetings and or more visible platforms, such as Facebook, where personal details, as well as contact with their offline friends was possible. This took great courage and trust, as often Stronger Together friends where brought in direct contact with the very people which the members would vent about in their journals and posts in a very open and disinhibited manner. However, for many the benefits of continuing these relationships far outweighed any possible problems. For example, in 2013, one member, after deciding to leave, contacts a number of her Stronger Together friends to let them know that she would be leaving and to ask them to join her as friends on Facebook. She opens her email by simply stating:

> It's just gotten too difficult. I need to start dealing with the reality of not being able to be pregnant …

Not wanting to sound ungrateful of the support received, she quickly moves on to assure her friends that:

> [H]onestly ST has been an amazing place for love and support the past two years and I have made lifelong friends who I will continue to keep in touch with …

After extensively discussing her reasons for leaving, she finally closes her email with the following:

> I am on Facebook if you want to look me up (Pam). You will see my wedding picture as my profile pic. A bunch of us from here started a private group on there to keep in touch and feel free to talk about IF or not to talk about it. Its actually nice to "see" the ladies in their NORMAL lives too! XOXO- Pam

For us, there were two particularly telling sections in the above email. First is the fact that Pam is incredibly concerned that her friends may think that she does not value their friendship, or sees their friendship as inferior and heads this by her statement "I have made lifelong friends ..." suggesting the genuineness of their bond, while simultaneously suggesting that their Stronger Together world falls somewhat outside the "norm" by stating that "It's actually nice to 'see' the ladies in their NORMAL lives too!" implying that moving into a more visual platform, such as Facebook, will allow friends to open a window into the "real" lives of members. In short, this farewell email, is a testament to the difficulties faced in online friendships, which while intense and very real, are also very tenuous. This vacillation may in part be due to the way in which support groups such as Stronger Together operate. As we have earlier shown in this section, for most of the participants, their support group required a very definite separation to offline interaction to maintain the appearance of anonymity and allow for disinhibited interaction. Bringing those who have been privy to some of their most intimate thoughts through the journey also meant the possibility of disclosure of aspects of their lives which some would rather remain hidden, such as intense episodes of venting. Yet, in the time in which we observed friendships that had moved outside the realm of Stronger Together it was clear that there seemed to be an innate understanding about the importance of discretion between Stronger Together members in these new social environments which allowed these friendships to continue to flourish.

It was not surprising to us that it was usually members who were ready to make the transition out of the group (due to either success or stopping treatment) that most often transitioned their friendships into the offline world. For these women, the need to maintain a neutral space in which to air the stresses of the journey was of less importance and this was instead replaced by a need to share their new journey with those who could understand their unique outlook.

Conclusion

For those facing the challenges of infertility, the friendships made in online support groups become an important source of support. As will be discussed in future chapters, these friendships become even more essential as offline relationships are destabilised by the infertility roller-coaster. As time progresses and these relationships become cemented, many of the women choose to move these friendships offline, and thus supplement their eroded face-to-face networks. For these women, the online environment is a haven; a place in which they can share their intimate thoughts, fears, sorrows and joys; find companionship and understanding and gather much needed emotional support. In short, for many, the communal spaces provided by OSGs such as Stronger Together make the lonely journey of infertility less isolating and more empowering.

References

Barak, A., Boniel-Nissim, M., & Suler, J. (2008). Fostering Empowerment in Online Support Groups. *Computers in Human Behavior, 24*(5), 1867–1883.

Bauman, Z. (2003). *Liquid Love: On the Frailty of Human Bonds.* Cambridge: Polity Press.

Beck, U., & Beck-Gernsheim, E. (1995). *The Normal Chaos of Love.* Oxford: Polity Press.

Campos-Castillo, C., & Hitlin, S. (2013). Copresence: Revisiting a Building Block for Social Interaction Theories. *Sociological Theory, 31*(2), 168–192.

Chambers, D. (2013). *Social Media and Personal Relationships: Online Intimacies and Personal Friendships.* Basingstoke: Palgrave Macmillan.

Dickerson, F. B. (1998). Strategies That Foster Empowerment. *Cognitive and Behavioral Practice, 5*(2), 255–275.

Giddens, A. (1992). *The Transformation of Intimacy: Sexuality, Love and Eroticism in Modern Societies.* Cambridge: Polity Press.

Groos, N. (2005). The Detraditionalization of Intimacy Reconsidered. *Sociological Theory, 23*(3), 286–311.

Hart, M. (2015). Youth Intimacy on Tumblr: A Pilot Study. *Young, 23*(3), 193–207.

Lapidot-Lefler, N., & Barak, A. (2015). The Benign Online Disinhibition Effect: Could Situational Factors Induce Self-Disclosure and Prosocial Behaviors? *Cyberpsychology: Journal of Psychosocial Research on Cyberspace, 9*(2), Article 3, 1–19.

Lieberman, M. A., & Goldstein, B. A. (2006). Not All Negative Emotions Are Equal: The Role of Emotional Expression in Online Support Groups for Women with Breast Cancer. *Psycho-Oncology, 15*(2), 160–168.

Suler, J. (2004). The Online Disinhibition Effect. *CyberPsychology & Behavior,* *7*(3), 321–326.

van Uden-Kraan, C. F., Drossaert, C. H. C., Taal, E., Seydel, E. R., & van Laar, M. A. F. (2008). Self-Reported Differences in Empowerment Between Lurkers and Posters in Online Patient Support Groups. *Journal of Medical Internet Research, 10*(2), e18.

4

A Glance in the Mirror: Women's Reflections on Their Emotions, Bodies and Selves

Anne-Maree Sawyer

'Why does this baby making business have to be so damn hard!?!?! I HOPE YOU ROT IN HELL, UNIVERSE!!!' (Sophie)
'Infertility has taken away the dream of what it means to get pregnant and feel excited about it ... Our struggle has become all we talk about, think about, save money for, cry about and dream about.' (Patricia)

Introduction

This chapter examines the women's accounts of how they experienced and managed their emotions, bodies and selves as they engaged in medical and non-medical treatments in an effort to achieve a "BFP" (Big Fat Positive). We focus here on their discursive practices—the particular language of selfhood and the frameworks of meaning the women used to make sense of, and deal with, situations that were often unpredictable and intensely distressing. As noted in Chap. 2, we envisage the online

A.-M. Sawyer (✉)
La Trobe University, Melbourne, Australia
e-mail: a.sawyer@latrobe.edu.au

© The Author(s) 2019
P. Billett, A.-M. Sawyer, *Infertility and Intimacy in an Online Community*,
Palgrave Macmillan Studies in Family and Intimate Life,
https://doi.org/10.1057/978-1-137-44981-8_4

support group as a very particular "narrative environment" (Gubrium 2005; Gubrium and Holstein 2009). The excerpts and exchanges from the women's journals and discussion boards discussed in this chapter, and throughout the book, demonstrate the common frameworks, or explanations, they used to construct, reflect on, and re-craft their own and fellow members' stories. We can see how participants were encouraged to "emplot" their experiences in specific ways (Ricoeur 1991). In the women's accounts of their emotions, bodies and selves, discourses of "positive thinking", and individual responsibility and "working" on the self, figured prominently. Additionally, the "roller-coaster ride" of the IVF journey and the experience of "biographical disruption" (Bury 1982) brought about by infertility were also significant themes.

Holstein and Gubrium's (2000) model of interpretive practice, centred on discursive practices and discourses-in-practice, provides a useful paradigm for conceptualising the women's use of particular discourses in their processes of meaning-making. Holstein and Gubrium (2000, p. 94) use the term "discourses-in-practice" to refer to the available systems of understanding, "the discursive possibilities for, and resources of, self construction at particular times and places". The women's discursive practices, their "linguistic actions" (p. 90)—that is, the "labor involved in [their] reality-building projects"—can be understood as shaped by broader discourses-in-practice but not determined by them. As Gubrium and Holstein (2000, p. 102) have argued, "the self emanates from the interplay among institutional demands, restraints, and resources, on the one hand, and biographically informed, self-constituting social actions, on the other."

Engaging in positive thinking and staying positive, even against the odds, seemed to be the main currency of exchange, advice and support in the online support group. All participants were involved, to a greater or lesser extent, in discourses and practices of positive thinking. They also engaged in a range of other practices to improve their health, explicitly to heighten their chances of falling pregnant and of "carrying" their babies to full term. In the main, this "work on the self" involved dieting and exercise regimes, and such allied health interventions as massage and acupuncture. We could say that the women engaged in a form of "reproductive asceticism" (Ettore 2002, p. 246), in their efforts to take full control and responsibility for monitoring, controlling and maintaining their bodies. Intense self-surveillance in health-promoting practices and day-to-day coping was evident in many of the journal excerpts and discussion board posts, as we will show. Sociologically, we can understand these processes of disciplining and regulating the mind and the body through the broader lens of individualisation and governmentality, concepts enlarged on below.

This chapter opens with an analysis of several discussion board posts to exemplify and illustrate the significance of "positive thinking" in the women's efforts to manage their distress at failing to fall pregnant. These posts also express the "roller-coaster" quality of the IF journey, the contingent nature of this "game of chance". Rapid transitions from success to failure, and back again, characterised these stories. Having set the scene, we then consider two other dimensions of positive thinking. The first we refer to as the "imperative" of positive thinking. Several of Sophie's journal entries exemplified this dimension very clearly. Without positive thinking, there is no hope, no reason to stay involved in the treatments; it remains the only way of harnessing hope amid despair. The second dimension concerns the "dark side" of positive thinking. Patricia's story shows how she railed against the pressure of it, akin to walking on a tightrope; the tension of trying to "stay positive" was often unbearable while dealing with repeated disappointments. We then turn to the women's practices of disciplining their bodies through diet and exercise and other interventions, thus demonstrating their emphasis on individual responsibility. Finally, we examine questions of identity that were raised by the women as they managed the emotional and bodily effects of IF treatments. Some women felt consumed by the seemingly endless round of treatments, the strictures imposed by the treatments, and the mental energy and commitment required by the "journey". It has "taken over my life", as one woman put it: hitherto familiar habits, preoccupations, and dreams having given way to an obsessive focus on IF and the myriad strategies to resolve it. Others felt pressed by an existentially oriented quest for meaning, to understand why infertility "had happened" to them. Questions concerning "who am I now?" and "who are we as a couple?" were at the heart of these posts.

Positive Thinking

To demonstrate the significance of positive thinking to the women's meaning-making processes, we provide a close reading of several selected discussion board posts. Questions of how to "stay positive" in negotiating the highs and lows of the IF journey were frequently posted to the discussion board. In the following thread, initiated by Bernadette, a newcomer to the site, who felt "emotionally exhausted" after two years of failed fertility treatments, responding participants encouraged coping strategies centred on maintaining "faith" and positivity. Bernadette noted that she and her husband had been "tirelessly" trying to conceive (TTC), having undergone a battery of fertility tests, and for several months she had been battling the nasty side-effects of acne and severe PMS from clomid (an oral medication used to stimulate ovulation). Now in her early thirties, Bernadette was very conscious of the "clock ticking", and the "next step" of their treatment journey was to be IVF. She was especially fearful of continued failure and the "shame spiral" that would engulf her if it were unsuccessful. She also highlighted the isolation she felt from her "super fertile friends", who could not relate to their anguish, hence her reaching out to others in the OSG.

In the manner of a genuinely aligned therapeutic exchange, Anne focused on each element of Bernadette's post, reflecting back and identifying with her emotions. First, she empathised with her "struggles" and isolation, establishing an early connection by affirming their "similar situations", avowing that it was very difficult to witness others "popping babies out easily". She then revealed that she, too, was "awaiting IVF", and that the "financial side" (of having to save up for treatment) had enabled her time to "accept that path" and to investigate IVF procedures so as to render them less daunting. She explained that there were "lots of videos" online to demonstrate "how to do the injections", together with other valuable advice. Anne admitted to feeling scared about IVF, too, but encouraged Bernadette to "find a bunch of 'things'" to keep her "happy and busy"; in effect, a means of staying positive and maintaining hope. Anne's identification with Bernadette's situation and her optimistic approach to her own circumstances—that the waiting time served to demystify IVF, a range of bodily practices (yoga, running and massage) were keeping her "happy" and "busy", and an IVF cycle in one's early 30s promised greater success than in later years—provided Bernadette with the tools to rethink her situation through more hopeful eyes. Anne's use of such linguistic constructions as "some people read" to stay busy, and "*we* are young … it may help *our* chances" (emphasis added) incorporated Bernadette into the online community, while embracing her as part of it. In micro-sociological terms, we can understand Anne's support as a form of collaborative interpersonal emotion management (Francis 1997; Hochschild 1979).

Garry, a "DH", also responded to Bernadette's post, explaining that he had gone through IF with his first wife, and eventually had two daughters. With these experiences behind him, he assumed that having children would be much easier in his second marriage. But this was not to be; he and his DW (Dear Wife) had already gone through "countless numbers of IUIs" and "spent thousands on fertility meds". Eventually, like others, they had to "face the IVF hurdle". He then revealed that they had recently received news of their pregnancy following an ER and ET. In words approximating a sense of evangelical zeal, Garry argued that, while the path ahead may "seem" interminable now, it is but a mirage: "you'll be amazed how quickly you'll reach the rainbow if you just have faith in the process." In effect, he claimed that one must *have faith* in the "process" of conventional treatment options—believe in it, surrender to it, and ultimately success will follow. In this "reality-building" project (Holstein and Gubrium 2000, p. 94), Garry emphasised individual responsibility—that one's thoughts and attitudes, not biological chance, ensure future success; thus the individual is arbiter of her future. Bernadette responded, drawing hope from these experiences—a counterpoint to those of her "super fertile friends". Fundamentally, this sharing of successful experiences after much anguish, together with the positive reframing of various circumstances, reinforced positive thinking as a trustworthy discursive practice—as *the only way* to deal effectively with the distress of IF. In the sequence of moves, recounted above (from Bernadette to Anne, onto Garry, and back to Bernadette) we see the production of emotional energy and the emotional entrainment of a "successful" interaction (Jasper 2014).

Jenny also weighed into the conversation, agreeing wholeheartedly with Garry, and asserting that if you surrender and "just" believe in the process, positive thinking will win out. She used her own experience as evidence, explaining how she had "tried and tried, hoped and prayed" for success, and it was only when she relaxed her efforts and "just believed that it would one day happen" that her prayers were answered. She proudly reported that she was now 16 weeks pregnant via IUI. By way of encouraging Bernadette, she acknowledged the abundant support provided by Stronger Together participants who "got it": the benefits of expressing one's sadness and despair, "venting" about family and friends, and gaining hope from others' successes. She concluded her post by admitting that she had "never" expected to be one of the lucky ones in a position to "give hope" to others. Jenny's happy news offered a beacon of hope to others—a testament to the wisdom of "letting go" and the power of positive thinking (believing "it would one day happen"), born out of despair and hopelessness.

In another thread, in which the initiator, Sue, sought "positive words or stories or tips", we see again claims about the benefits of positive thinking. Having experienced a miscarriage, Sue worried about another failure and wanted to deal with her anxieties more effectively as she faced a frozen embryo transfer (FET) cycle. On the positive side of the ledger, she told herself that the miscarriage had demonstrated she was capable of falling pregnant. This time, for the FET cycle, she intended to "stay more calm" and "not stress", since she had been very "uptight" in the period leading into the miscarriage. Like other women on the site, she implied that her stressed state had contributed to, or even caused, the loss of the pregnancy. In this context, she asked for "positive words or stories or tips" to facilitate her resolve to stay positive. Utilising this particular logic of support seeking, Sue and other women on the site constructed themselves as enterprising individuals—reflexive health entrepreneurs—"willing and able to manage their own wellbeing" (Crawshaw 2012, p. 200). The women's online reflections on managing their emotions, bodies and selves, illustrates the way in which they had internalised the edicts of neo-liberal rationality, which "calls upon each of us to enter into the process of his or her own self governance through endless self examination, self care and self improvement" (Petersen 1996, p. 194). While this mode of problem-solving is potentially empowering (Barak et al. 2008), it may also become deeply demoralising when one's efforts are not rewarded.

Rebecca was also "gearing up" for FET. She empathised with Sue over the difficulty of remaining optimistic despite repeated failures, revealing that she had undergone several FET procedures resulting in a "chemical pregnancy" on the first attempt, followed by several miscarriages in later attempts. With each FET intervention she had tried not to raise her hopes because "I fear for the worst"; at the same time, she wanted to "be positive" because she believed it would ease "the whole mentality of everything"—that it would make her better able to deal with the wider emotional aspects of the IF journey. Barbara, also contributing to the thread, provided very strong testimony for the benefits of "staying as calm as possible" and "positive", drawing on experiences with a particular acupuncturist. She described herself as having been "a basket case" during an earlier failed IVF cycle, replete with high levels of stress and "negative thoughts" of failure. Not long afterwards, she "tried" a new acupuncturist, who told her she was "not ready" to have a baby. Though initially very perturbed by this assertively voiced opinion, Barbara saw its wisdom after the failure of a subsequent IVF cycle. She then moved onto donor eggs, and with the acupuncturist's treatments and guidance she donned a "very different attitude", claiming that the practitioner had "changed" her into "a different person—very calm and positive". After transfer, she "didn't google stuff". Instead, she "kept busy" and avoided reading meaning "into every little symptom." At the time of posting, Barbara was 15 weeks pregnant and claimed that "a huge part" of her success was due to the acupuncture and her new-found capacity to "stay calm". Drawing on empirical research, health sociologist Alex Broom (2009) argued that the appeal of complementary and alternative medicine seems rooted in its valuing of subjective experiences, the fostering of self-determination and empowerment, and the recovery of hope (see also Broom and Tovey 2007). These features characterised Barbara's portrayal of her interactions with the acupuncturist, whom she saw as possessing crucial intuitive insights into her personal needs and IF journey. In the conversational moves from Sue to Rebecca and onto Barbara, we see again the progressive development of views about the significance of positive thinking and individualised responsibility for wellbeing, each building on and reinforcing the other's account in a process of collaborative "reality-building" (Holstein and Gubrium 2000, p. 94).

The Imperative of Positive Thinking

Although Sophie played with the practice of positive thinking in a humorous and, perhaps, ironic manner, her efforts seemed at once to both mask and reveal the imperative of positive thinking in the endeavour of "TTC". Without it there could be no hope, no door opened to future possibilities of success. Yet, as most of the women showed in their posts, positive thinking was a buffer against the hard realities of their situations, the unknown futures—evoked in the oft-cited refrain that perhaps there will be another chance, no matter how slim.

In her first journal entry, Sophie reported that she had recently "lost a pregnancy" but no longer allowed herself to "feel completely devastated by it". Rather, adopting a partly serious/partly comic proclivity she demonstrated the significance of positive thinking, noting that she had been "feeling really optimistic lately" and explaining how she worked to produce this particular self-construction:

> My coping strategy seems to be the 'looking toward the future' kind. I allow myself to think of the lost baby but I don't allow myself to feel completely devastated by it anymore. I haven't figured out if that's a good or bad thing, but right now I'm just enjoying the peace of mind. I think I have successfully convinced myself that the lost baby only made my body more fertile so the next batch of eggs I produce is going to be top-notch! I'm going to produce a wonder child, isn't that great?!

Sophie then revealed, tongue-in-cheek, that she had been trying to come up with a "list of positives to this infertility/IVF situation" but thus far could think of only one—"but it's a good one":

> When my IVF conceived child is a sarcastic cynical teenager giving me hell about not going to the movies on a school night, I will get to say, 'Look, if you don't stop sassing me, I will quit making payments on you and you will get repo'd!'

A few days later, frustrated and upset over miscommunications from two professionals in her treating team as she and her husband planned their second IVF cycle, Sophie embraced the imperative of positive thinking. A nurse had told them they could start the next cycle in May "as long as we were emotionally ready". Eventually this did happen but in the midst of confused messages from the two professionals, she posted:

> Are you F#@*ing kidding me? WHY was I told that a May cycle was possible then? WHY would you allow me to plan for a whole week and get my hopes up? OHMYGOD this just pisses me off to no end. GET YOUR S@#* TOGETHER AND QUIT MESSING WITH MY LIFE!

Then, engaging in active emotion regulation, she explained:

> Ok, now that my rant is over, I need to throw in a positive or else I'll suffocate in negative feelings: We were invited to be a part of a Murder Mystery Dinner in July at an old 'haunted' hotel, but the hubby and I weren't sure about it since it was possible we could have been about 10 weeks pregnant. Well now, I am definitely doing it and I'm excited!

Two months on from her first journal entry, Sophie announced to the group that she was pregnant, officially. (This pregnancy would result in two healthy boys.) Again, the emphasis was on positive thinking and her consciousness of struggling "very hard" to maintain it: "I am trying very hard to relish in this moment and enjoy this time but it's very hard! I keep worrying about the worst but then I force myself to think happy positive thoughts. I need to stay optimistic for this baby!" She then revealed a self-disciplining strategy she had settled upon to achieve this, echoing the resolves made by some of the other women on the site:

> I am definitely going to stop researching the internet and looking at other people's stories. Just because it happened to them doesn't mean it's going to happen to me. I am going to read my *What to Expect when you're Expecting* book and only research good happy pregnant things!

Nevertheless, as numerous posts to the general discussion board demonstrated, many of the women found it excruciatingly difficult to sustain positive thoughts after the heartbreak of losing a seemingly healthy

pregnancy that had followed sustained, multiple failures. Daphne's situation was not unusual. She opened her post by explaining why she had
been absent from the site for some 12 months: after several unsuccessful
IUIs, she had fallen pregnant on the next one. It was "the happiest time
ever" for Daphne and her husband. Alas, when attending a follow-up
appointment, they discovered that their "little boy had passed away at 7
weeks": a harrowing experience, since they had "seen and heard the heart-
beat". Subsequent IUI attempts were unsuccessful, although promising
in the early stages. The next step was IVF, "totally new" to them and
daunting because it was not covered by health insurance (costing over
$10,000) and their "last chance" for a baby. Daphne admitted she was
"scared" about her unknown future. Maggie responded very empathically, posting that IVF was "stressful", "expensive" and "time-consum-
ing", and expressed hope that Daphne's first IVF cycle would bring
success. In spite of Daphne's litany of failures, Maggie doggedly asserted
the imperative of staying positive, urging that such interventions as IVF
were their "only hope" and "we just have to keep believing that it will
work." Claims about the need to stay positive and "keep believing" were
thus encouraged in the narrative environment of Stronger Together.
Beyond such offerings, there seemed little else in the way of emotional
resources that the women could draw on in supporting one another.

The "Dark Side" of Positive Thinking

In this section, we focus primarily on Patricia's story. Her journal entries
stand out because she elucidated very clearly the pressure of trying to
maintain a positive outlook in the face of repeated disappointments. In
some of her entries, she "spoke back" to the burden of staying positive,
railing against it and giving vent to her anger and frustration. When
Patricia commenced her journal, she and her husband were in their early
40s, and poised to embark on their second IVF attempt. Patricia continued recording their experiences in her journal through several further
IVF and IUI attempts over the following years. She was acutely conscious
of the prevailing influence that positive thinking played in "framing" and
"doing matters of relevance" to group members (Gubrium 2005, p. 526).

In an early journal entry, facing her second IUI, she revealed her struggle to adopt a positive stance:

It is so hard to be positive *like everyone says I need to be* because I am so worried about the HUGE letdown if it doesn't work. It is so much easier to prepare myself in advance for disappointment. I am going to try my best to stay positive this time! Maybe the distraction of the first two weeks of school is a good thing! I will be thinking about it less and exhausted at the end of the day to dwell on anything BUT school and my new students.

Lizzie supported the strategy Patricia had identified as a means of avoiding negativity and despair while waiting, thus reinforcing the discourse of positivity, and agreeing that the busyness of a new school year "will be *a good thing*" (our emphasis). She also identified deeply with Patricia, revealing that she, too, was "going nuts" with the stress of waiting to find out if her procedure had worked. Concluding her brief message in a very easy-going, conversational tone with "I am rooting for you!" and "Keep me posted" imparted further reassurance to Patricia to "stay positive". These words signified that *we are in this together and what you feel is important, so let me know what happens.* Such affecting words act to produce an intimate bond, an emotional connection in the online space (Hinton et al. 2010).

Some two months on, following her third IUI, planned initially as an IVF cycle, Patricia again revealed the difficulty of staying positive amid failure:

It's official—third round of IUI (should have been IVF but only produced one egg) and another BFN! They don't get easier to hear! I feel defeated and so sad! I don't know how much more I have in me! Getting up at 5am today to go out into the dark and cold to be at the RE for a 6.30am appointment so I can make it to work in time for my class to show up is exhausting and all I see ahead are many more dark and cold mornings with snow and cleaning it off my car ... ugh! I just don't know how to get positive about all those meds and what they are NOT doing for me.

Patricia's beseechingly honest presentation of her feelings seemed to beg the question of how one might "do" positive thinking, given these circumstances, when "all" she could "see ahead" were the "exhausting" routines on "dark and cold mornings", and the unremitting demands of her full-time teaching job.

Seven months later, amid the failure of her third IVF treatment and the lead up to the next attempt, Patricia questioned the utility of positive thinking as an emotional coping strategy, especially in light of the irrefutable fact of biology. She prefaced her post with an apology ("I hate to say this"), an acknowledgement that she was letting the side down, deviating from the normative script:

> I hate to say this, but the power of positivity is being lost on me. I see all of you wonderful women on here getting your BFP and I just don't understand why it is so hard for me to get a piece of that luck/joy. I am panicking that we are near our end of trying. Insurance money is running out. DH is still not working (he left his job to work on a start-up company that is not making any money yet and we don't know when/if it will) so we cannot afford to pay out of pocket after the insurance money runs out. I am 42 (DH is 47) so biologically our days are numbered.

In this excerpt, Patricia lifted the lid on the fraudulent nature of positive thinking, while admitting and apologising for her failure to self-regulate.

As she approached her fourth IVF cycle, Patricia sought to trust in the promise of positive thinking, to align herself with the lore of the group, but was "nervous" of being cheated by another failure:

> Want to be more positive, but it makes me so nervous to be that hopeful! The changes in this cycle compared to the previous ones seem like a good sign, but until I see my stomach growing larger for reasons other than the weight gain from stims I am not sure if I can believe that this will work! I know I need to believe (and secretly I think I do) but so scared to admit it out loud!

Here Patricia articulated the turmoil of the emotional "roller-coaster"—akin to walking along an emotional precipice—a very common experience expressed by the women of Stronger Together. At a more abstract level, the excerpt shows very poignantly the inner work of self-monitoring and self-surveillance, while grappling with fear.

Patricia fell pregnant eventually. In the first few weeks, she felt very tentative about the future of the pregnancy and admitted her failure to feel positive:

> So I should be sitting here happy as can be because I AM PREGNANT! Instead I am panicked because I know we are not out of the woods. We still haven't seen our baby on a sono and we have no idea what tomorrow's sono will bring. I still can't wrap my head around the fact that I am indeed pregnant. I continue to say things like, 'If we have a baby next year' or 'If I'm still pregnant.' I know, it's negative thinking but I am scared shitless right now.

Sadly, there were "abnormalities" and the foetus did not develop. Patricia was forced to have a "D & C", which was "devastating".

Another three months on, she was ready to start her fifth IVF cycle, following a rough few months characterised by increased "stressful" work demands, physical health problems unrelated to infertility, and "a ton of doctors' appointments". Despite the disappointments endured thus far, Patricia expressed a strong commitment to renew her investment in positive thinking ("to push myself to believe"):

> I still cannot believe I am doing this again! IVF #5. I am going to try my best to believe and send only positive thoughts out into the universe for this cycle. It's so easy to NOT believe and think negatively ... it comes naturally to me at this point after so much disappointment, but I am going to push myself to believe.

Patricia's emphasis on individual responsibility was palpable, carrying the conviction that *I can be positive if only I try hard enough*. However, with "poor results on the stims" only two eggs were produced, so "what should have been IVF #5 ... turned into IUI #5." Three months later, Patricia decided to try IVF again; it was unsuccessful (three out of four eggs fertilised and were transferred) and five days later she used a home pregnancy test:

I did the ultimate NO-NO today and took a HPT because my intuition tells me I am not going to be pregnant this time. I am just going to be fat, bruised and feeling down so start preparing for the spiral downward once again. Of course the HPT said BFN and confirmed how I was feeling.

The three days later (and seven days post-ET), Patricia protested against positive thinking as a self-management practice, distancing herself from those who argued that "faith" and "positivity" would bring results:

> Now I know that some people feel 'She's just so negative' and 'Of course, it won't happen if you don't believe' … After so many crushing blows (seriously I believe I have peed on NO JOKE at LEAST 50-60 HPT in the past 2 years) how on EARTH am I supposed to remain positive and hopeful? I go into the cycle feeling good, midway I freak out a bit, and then I have the transfer and I feel hopeful again, only to be let down time and time again. And I know many of you have felt this way too after dealing with IF for as long, if not longer than I have. And maybe your 'faith' and 'positivity' are what you feel will make it work for you … and I HOPE YOU ARE RIGHT!

In a similar vein to Patricia, Kate, introduced in Chap. 2, "spoke back" to the discourse of positive thinking in a post to the general discussion board. After more than seven IUI and IVF cycles, she confessed she "had to stop trying" in order to prevent bankruptcy and to "save" her marriage. For now, at least, Kate had reached the end of the road, and saw the insistence on positive thinking as a curse rather than a form of deliverance. In an emotive plea, she requested that others on the site refrain from posting comments insisting that "it will happen" because she knew "for a fact that it will not." With what remained from years of "no luck", she was working "very hard" to accept the loss of her dreams and "make peace" with "the Universe".

Kate's post placed her outside the going concerns of the OSG. She received no responses. She had asked that her narrative not be "repaired" (Gubrium 2005, p. 526) and, in refusing the dominant frame of positive thinking, there was no story for a potential respondent to offer within the narrative environment of Stronger Together. Kate's post presents a heart-rending picture of infertility as a form of "disenfranchised" grief (Doka

1989, 2002), an experience of loss and sorrow that is not readily socially recognised. There are no culturally prescribed guidelines in which people can engage to mourn the loss of their hopes and expectations of "having a family".

Patricia's journal excerpts provide moving insights into the felt pressure to "stay positive", regardless of one's reproductive circumstances and history. Patricia shines a light on the unrealistic, hoax-like aspects of positive thinking as a means of attaining success, while also accepting it as the main currency of exchange in the online interactions and, at times, apologising for her struggles to embrace it. In this way, she did her own "repair" work, policing her capacities to conform to the discourse of positive thinking (Gubrium 2005). With mounting failures, she questioned its utility more forcefully and finally admitted "after so many crushing blows" that she could not make it "work" for her. Kate, on the other hand, yearned to "make peace", to adjust to the reality of her failed attempts to have a family. Messages of positivity and assurances of success could have no place in the new narrative she was striving to forge for herself. Without culturally prescribed guides of how to live beyond the failures wrought by infertility treatments, each woman must fall back on her own resources to create "peace" and meaning (Beck and Beck-Gernsheim 2002). The promise held out by assisted reproductive technologies (ARTs) has enabled some women to "re-invent" their lives, to embrace the culturally normative narrative of motherhood. Yet, women for whom ART has not been successful, women who have reached the end of the "journey", are likely to remain bereft of publicly available narratives to guide them into the future (Leigh 2016). If we accept that people live by stories (Bruner 1987; Holstein and Gubrium 2000; May 2012; Richardson 1990)—and if the narratives available at a particular socio-cultural moment are out of step with some people's lived experiences—then, their lives may "end up being limited and textually disenfranchised" (Richardson 1990, p. 129).

In historical terms, women for whom ARTs have not been successful constitute a relatively new group in the population, and narratives have not yet evolved to reflect and address the very particular social and personal experiences of involuntary childlessness following failed IF treatments. In much the same way as published autobiographies and identity politics fostered widespread consciousness of the social suffering of same-sex attracted people, African-Americans, Indigenous peoples and other minorities in the late twentieth century, so too, published accounts of women's experiences of failed IF treatments are needed as cultural guides or templates—to give voice to their very particular, untold experiences of suffering. New narratives are required to accommodate the socio-emotional circumstances produced by (failed) infertility treatments, to guide and heal women to live beyond these experiences, so that the "story of a transformed life ... becomes a part of the cultural heritage affecting future stories and future lives" (Richardson 1990, p. 129; see also Saleebey 1994; Wilkinson and Kleinman 2016). While personal stories of depression, grief, and cancer (e.g. Didion 2005; Hitchens 2012; Lewis 1961; Lourde 1980; Styron 1990; Wurtzel 1994) are well established in the public sphere as sub-genres of the illness narrative, stories of infertility are not. Julia Leigh's (2016) recent memoir of IVF, *Avalanche*, is a rare exception. Illness narratives, published as fiction, biography and autobiography, generate societal as well as therapeutic benefits. Textual representations of experience have the potential to generate sympathy and understanding, reduce the stigma associated with illnesses, and offer models of how to live through and beyond a particular illness (Frank 2010; Richardson 1990).

Disciplining the Body (and the Mind)

In an effort to maximise their health—and thus their chances of falling pregnant—many of the women engaged in specific practices of self-care and self-regulation, most often through diet and exercise. Sociologically, we can understand the broader context of these efforts with reference to the concepts of risk, individualisation, and governmentality. Beck's (1992) seminal "risk society" thesis is pertinent to situating the women's infertile bodies in contemporary discourses and health-care practices. As Beck and others (e.g. Giddens 1991; Lupton 2013) have argued, risk consciousness is pervasive in everyday life. The rise of risk consciousness is related, in part, to processes of individualisation; traditional guides and routines that previously structured the life-course have given way to an emphasis on reflexivity and individuality, now central defining features of contemporary life. Our lives have become disembedded from the shaping influences of class, gender, ethnicity and community, which no longer determine our biographical paths to the same extent as in the past. As a consequence, we have more freedom to "write" our own biographies, to author our identities by choosing from an array of possibilities (Giddens 1991). While choice is liberating, it also produces insecurity and a burden on individual responsibility. The spectre of risk is ever-present: the risk of making the wrong choice, of trusting the wrong expert. In an era in which experts and expert knowledge are no longer seen as infallible—coupled with the increasing influence of consumer health movements and the plethora of information available on the Internet—individuals are required to reflexively sift through and assess the knowledge at hand. The downside of individualisation, as Lupton (2012, p. 331) has argued, is that "people are blamed for making the wrong choices when things go wrong in their lives." Posting about their self-care practices, the women of Stronger Together frequently blamed themselves for failing to maintain what were seemingly very arduous regimes.

A further interpretive lens relevant to the women's self-care practices concerns the Foucauldian related concepts of the "neoliberal government" of citizens and "biopolitics" (Lupton 2012). In neoliberal regimes:

> [C]itizens are expected to take responsibility for their own actions and welfare ... to voluntarily position themselves as responsible for themselves, to monitor, regulate and discipline their own bodies in their own interest ...
>
> Foucault's concept of biopolitics is related to neoliberalism. Biopolitics refers to the apparatuses of expert knowledge and practice which represent and discipline human embodiment ... All citizens in modern neoliberal societies are made aware of their responsibilities to conform to expert advice concerning the monitoring, regulation and disciplining of their bodies. Health promotion, medical testing regimes and public health activities are all agents of the government of citizens' health. The management of the health of one's body has become a feature of good citizenship, a dimension of the 'care of the self'. (Lupton 2012, p. 335)

Hence, in terms of biopolitics, governing the self involves an "ethical responsibility" (Lupton 2012, p. 336) to keep abreast of the latest relevant

health information, to seek and weigh up expert opinions, and to utilise biomedical interventions and those offered by complementary and
alternative medicine. Erin's journal is a case in point. Many of her
entries focused on bodily and emotional self-care practices in the manner of a reflexive health entrepreneur (Crawshaw 2012, p. 200)—diet,
exercise, acupuncture, sleep and relaxation, and generally managing
her health. Her very organised and holistic approach was probably
shaped by her particular orientation to health and wellbeing as a case
manager in a mental health service. Our occupations shape our identities and lives, providing a "recognized means of characterizing and
making sense of things, including important ways of accounting for
oneself and others … with what amounts to a set of interpretive tools
for making meaning" (Gubrium and Holstein 2009, p. 161). Erin
seemed to self-manage along the lines of how she might reasonably
have expected her clients to exercise "good citizenship" in approaching
their own self-care.

She often "reported in" to the Stronger Together group, giving updates
on the progress of her goals, and noting the additional "work" needed to
achieve them, as demonstrated in an early journal entry: "The diet is
going well so far. I find that I can easily be strict during the week about
it, and I 'take a break' on weekends, which means that I still try not to go
crazy, but I don't worry about making sure that everything I put in my
mouth is on the green list. So far, I have lost a couple of pounds, which
is good considering I still haven't gotten into an exercise routine."

Two weeks later, she made another entry about her diet, focusing on
the minutiae of her experiences. Here she used her journal as a vehicle for
self-monitoring and motivation, reflecting on the factors that enabled her
to meet her goals:

> I have definitely noticed a difference in my moods and appetite since I
> started this diet. Today begins week 4 and I no longer feel like a slave to
> food. I used to be so depressed and ate when I was bored, stressed, excited,
> etc. Now, it is more just something I do. Sometimes, I almost dread it
> because I don't feel hungry most of the time, but I know I need to maintain
> pretty steady sugar levels. What a great feeling it is! I forgot what it was like
> to not feel like a food addict!

In another journal entry, Erin gave an expanded account of the range of strategies in which she had invested, demonstrating her "ethical responsibility" (Lupton 2012, p. 336) in considering a piece of expert advice she had recently "heard" about:

> I found some new diabetic supplements that are designed for diabetics. Although I'm not a diabetic, I have a family history of this and since I have PCOS, I figured I would give these vitamins a try. They happen to include all the vitamins I have heard are helpful anyway. I ordered Vitex last week and it should arrive any day. I am so excited to start taking it!
>
> I plan to call this week to schedule an appointment with a new family doctor ... Still looking for a new OBGYN that has privileges at the hospital I like ...
>
> I have been exercising a little more (though I could certainly improve in that area). I bought and am using a pedometer to make sure that I at least do something more than the minimum every day.

Of the complementary and alternative therapies discussed by Stronger Together participants, acupuncture was mentioned most. These therapies seemed to hold out much promise, according to reports from the women who had used them and claims made by therapists themselves, as shown in the following excerpts from Erin's journal:

> I'm seeing my acupuncturist on Friday and I'm hoping she can help my body get back to where it should be. I'm really excited and hopeful that it helps!

A few days later she described her first acupuncture treatment:

> My acupuncturist is very confident that I will get pregnant with this treatment. I told her that I have been on Metformin and am getting ready to start Clomid and she thinks that my medications along with acupuncture are definitely going to do the trick for me ... there was no doubt in her voice and she said it pretty matter-of-factly. I sure hope she is right.
>
> The experience itself was pretty cool. I haven't really noticed a difference in how I feel or anything yet, but she talked about how my energy is 'stuck', especially on my left side. After she put the needles in, she checked again and said she could feel the difference and was sure that with more treatment, everything would get back to where it needs to be.

A week later, Erin noted again the acupuncturist's confidence in the treatment:

> I'm continuing acupuncture for the moment. I don't notice a difference, but my acupuncturist is confident that this will help and that we'll get pregnant in no time. I hope she's right. I will keep it going for at least another month or two, while I start treatment with an RE.

In contrast with Erin, some women took up complementary and alternative therapies because they felt pressured to do so by their primary treating practitioners and by others. Patricia's doctor encouraged her to "do" acupuncture: "She swears she has had a lot of successful results when using it. The problem is that I don't know how much I believe in it AND it is not covered … by my insurance."

Reporting on her first acupuncture treatment, Patricia questioned the practitioner's assessment of her health, envisaging the stress and anxiety of yet another disciplinary practice she realised she would feel compelled to follow:

> I had the WORST day. My DH took me to the acupuncturist … We discussed my diet (which I never thought was bad … I don't drink caffeinated stuff, I don't eat anything fried, I don't eat junk food on a regular basis, etc.). Apparently she believes I suffer from fibroids because I eat dairy (and not even much of that … I have a bowl of cereal for breakfast and a piece of cheese during the day … every so often we have pizza). She wants me to change my diet … no dairy, more fruit (which I really don't like), veggies (which I eat a lot of) … better chicken (more organic etc.) … Then she thinks I have to start fish oil and some herbal crap. Telling me all of that made me so stressed out! As if I don't have enough to think about, and FUNCTION NORMALLY for work on a daily basis, now I have to be worried that I am not eating correctly, when all along I didn't think I was bad at all.

New practices demanded new and heightened forms of self-surveillance which, in Patricia's case, seemed to reach into almost every facet of her everyday life.

The women of Stronger Together also posted about the difficulties they had in maintaining various self-imposed bodily regimes. Some posts were self-chastising in tone, while others provided a very detailed picture of the ups and downs of sticking to specific routines. In writing these accounts the women provided themselves with an explanation of their progress, thereby setting their self-care practices and bodily activities in the broader narrative context of their "IF journey". The following two excerpts from Joan's journal illustrate this process. She described herself as having "a mixed bag of anxiety and depression", along with infertility, and focused on the need to lose weight through exercise and dieting. In the first of these journal excerpts, she revealed her struggle to stay motivated in the quest to lose a significant amount of weight. It seemed very likely that the online space enabled her revelation of these deeply personal details that may otherwise have been too embarrassing or distressing to disclose in a face-to-face support-seeking setting (Barak et al. 2008; Singleton et al. 2016; White and Dorman 2001):

> [M]y mood has plummeted and I'm no longer caring about riding my bike or doing anything to lose the excess weight I have. I'm not one to be embarrassed about my weight, so I'll go ahead and say it up front. I'm fat. Morbidly obese according to my doctors. My BMI is at 49, I'm two times the size of a 'typical' woman my height. I'm 5 foot 4 inches tall and weigh 285 pounds (roughly, haven't weighed myself in the past week). I need to lose *at least* 130 pounds to be in my 'healthy' range. I'm currently hoping I can somehow muster the motivation to at least lose 85 and get down to 200 pounds by next summer.
>
> I just can't find anything that motivates me. I even tried the whole 'my chances of getting pregnant increase as I lose weight' spiel, but it didn't even work. I don't know how to keep myself motivated. My DH keeps trying, bless him, to help me find something to motivate me and keep me moving, but nothing either of us has tried has helped.

Some twelve months later, with the same weight loss goal, Joan tried a different tack. Rather than the self-talk of her earlier (failed) attempt, she turned to a website tracker to help her "track" her "calorie differential" on a daily basis. By taking "one step at a time" she hoped to preserve her motivation to lose 200 pounds over two years:

I'm down another pound, which means I'm in all down 3 pounds since I started this whole thing almost a month ago. 3 pounds is a very good start. Last time I tried to lose weight, I only logged/monitored my weight once per month, so I saw an overall number that was large. It kept me going for a while, but eventually when the number started getting smaller, I lost motivation. Hopefully watching the weight come off, pound by pound, week by week, will keep me motivated to keep up with the weight loss/ work outs.

Using a website to track my calorie intake and calories burned showed me that for now, I barely have to do anything to get the pound per week off. A book I read told me that 3,500 calories is the equivalent of one pound. So, if I make sure my calorie differential (burned vs eaten) is at -500 per day, I'll lose a pound a week. Seems hard to keep track of, but the website (if you use it every day) tracks it for you. I found out that adding 20 minutes of walking actually equals that -500 differential number I'm looking for.

I'll obviously have to keep changing my daily calorie allowance as I lose more and more weight, so I'll have to keep changing my workouts too … Losing weight will help on my IF journey for many reasons, the most important of which is qualifying for IVF once I reach my goal weight! I've given myself 2 years to get to 200 pounds (where my BMI will be just under 35), so that I have a chance to get there without going 'Well, I didn't make it …' at the end of the year and feeling like crap and losing motivation. I'm hoping once the summer gets here that I can increase my weight loss to two pounds per week.

… In the summer I'll have an outdoor pool to swim in on the really hot days. And come the fall I'll have access to a gym at the college when I start my courses. Now to get over the embarrassment I feel in a gym … oh well, one step at a time!

Erin's investment in a pedometer and Joan's use of a website tracker exemplifies how their self-care practices intersected with broader consumer culture. These participants, along with many others from the OSG, looked to the market for solutions to personal problems—a key characteristic of late western modernity (Beck and Beck-Gernsheim 2002; Crawshaw 2012; Giddens 1991). As "good" citizens, they assumed responsibility for their welfare by voluntarily positioning themselves "to monitor, regulate and discipline their own bodies in their own interest"

(Lupton 2012, p. 335). Hence, exercise equipment companies and those creating software to track individuals' physiological data constitute "agents of the government of citizens' health" (Lupton 2012, p. 335).

In the excerpts discussed above, we see the cultural logics of neoliberalism writ large—above all, looking first to the self (Silva 2013, p. 14). "Good" citizenship in late modernity is achieved by managing the self, taking care of one's health, as argued above. For women who are infertile, this means dieting, exercising, "doing" acupuncture, and undergoing the gamut of medical interventions provided by fertility clinics; that is, engaging in biopolitics: making use of "the apparatuses of expert knowledge and practice which represent and discipline human embodiment" (Lupton 2012, p. 335).

Fertility treatments are costly, financially, emotionally and physically; but the hope of forming a family, often intensified by the claims of fertility clinics, drives many couples to endure the hardships of treatment—sometimes for years at a time, as evidenced by many of the journal entries and posts on the Stronger Together site. Yet, the success of treatment is relatively low, with success rates often exaggerated. A recent episode of *Four Corners* (ABC TV 2016), Australia's leading investigative journalism programme, revealed that the industry's multi-million dollar profits are being protected at the expense of providing accurate data on the chances of "success" (live births):

> **Professor Gab Kovacs, former director of Monash IVF:** 'The chance of success by IVF is, by far, best dependant on your age ... and it starts going downhill from 35 onwards. We're using a medical treatment for a social problem. We need to educate a population that you're meant to have children in your early 30s, not in your early 40's.'
>
> **Sarah Dingle, reporter:** 'The reality is: what's being sold to women in their 40s is often false hope. Based on figures provided by the industry, a 43-year-old Australian woman, using her own 43-year-old eggs to conceive, has less than a three per cent chance of going home with a live baby. Put another way: she has a more than 97 per cent chance of failure every time.'

Professor Alan Trounson, another scientist and Australian IVF pioneer, interviewed by *Four Corners*, argued that the IVF clinics were generally not "transparent" in providing patients with "understandable" statistics showing the probability of achieving a live birth (ABC TV 2016). As a consequence of the commercialisation of the IVF industry, increased numbers of treatment cycles mean greater profits for these corporations. Given such low rates of success for women in their 40s—the fastest growing group receiving IVF treatments—could we claim that these corporations are selling "false hope"? (ABC TV 2016) In this context, Julia Leigh, also interviewed for this programme, explained that, "We're often hearing the success stories … in fact, I can't think of many stories of IVF failure out there." If the dominant narrative associated with IVF concerns the miracle of an individual woman's eventual "success" in the (neoliberal) ideological setting of free choice and individual responsibility, other ways of understanding the situation are thus obscured. Furthermore, if fertility clinics *are* "selling" hope, how does a women decide when to stop trying, especially when the desire to "carry your own child" is "so strong" and when she has the "freedom" to choose another cycle of treatment (ABC TV 2016)? What if the next cycle brings success, even against miniscule odds? Accordingly, the *imperative* of positive thinking, discussed above, echoed in the words of Julia Leigh: "An IVF patient is living and breathing hope … You wouldn't do it if you didn't have a sense of hope. Why would you put yourself through it?" (ABC TV 2016).

As we have shown in this chapter, the narrative environment of Stronger Together encouraged individualised stories of "positive thinking" and "working" on the self. Broader issues, such as IVF success rates, and "bigger picture" views concerning the commercialisation of fertility interventions were discouraged. Of all the posts and online journal entries we examined, Patricia was the only participant who seemed open to some of these "bigger" issues—open to questioning or critiquing what the experts said. We see this in her approach to positive thinking and to the facts of biology. Strikingly, other participants on the site did not engage with these facets of her posts; instead, they empathised with her sadness and distress, and encouraged her to "stay positive": therapeutic responses that stayed clear of the (broader) structural arrangements that shape women's IF journeys. Rather, as we have shown, the women's identities were grounded in their capacities to give voice to the minutiae of their emotional ups and downs, their capacities to self-regulate, and the conduct of individualised healthcare practices. Inspired by the work of Jennifer Silva

(2013) and Eva Illouz (2008), we might argue that the women made meaning out of emotional self-management and wilful self-change, the cultural logics entailed in the therapeutic narrative of selfhood. In the same way that the market economy compels individuals to continually monitor, discipline and transform their bodies in order to maximise their health in their own interests (Crawshaw 2012; Lupton 2012), therapeutic culture requires "vigilant self-monitoring and transformation in the emotional sphere in order to achieve happiness and wellbeing" (Silva 2013, p. 12; see Illouz 2008). The therapeutic narrative "provides a blueprint for bringing a reconstructed, healthy self into being":

> Inwardly directed and preoccupied with its own psychic and emotional growth, the therapeutic self has become a crucial cultural resource for ascribing meaning and order to one's life amid the flux and uncertainty of a flexible economy and a post-traditional social world. (Silva 2013, p. 19)

Neoliberalism and biopolitical frames foster the idea that people are responsible for their economic wellbeing and their health, and therapy culture "renders them responsible for their *emotional* fates" (Silva 2013, p. 21; italics included). The Stronger Together posts examined thus far, and in subsequent chapters, illustrate how the interrelated influences of neoliberalism and therapy culture were woven into the women's discursive practices in the online space. Malik and Coulson's (2010) finding that "support or empathy" and the "sharing of personal experiences" were, overwhelmingly, the most frequently used self-help mechanisms in a UK-based OSG, as noted in Chap. 2, also illustrates the pervasiveness of the therapeutic narrative as a cultural resource "for ascribing meaning and order to one's life" (Silva 2013, p. 19; see Illouz 2003, 2008).

Existential Anxiety and Questions of Identity: Who Am I Now?

Not surprisingly, the ongoing experience of infertility with its ups and downs called into question the women's experiences of their own identities. Many felt that their "infertile" status had taken over their identities, that their preoccupations and activities were almost completely focused on dealing with IF, often to the detriment of their health, relationships, interests and employment. Some of the women conveyed a sense of being out of control, especially when attempting to negotiate sudden shifts between the promise of success and the heartbreak of failure, referred to as the "roller-coaster ride". At times, there were no words to adequately describe the feelings of despair and bodily disarray, as Patricia declared in a journal entry:

> I can't even begin to explain how devastated I feel. My body is failing me … my mind is failing me … I am so scattered, lack of sleep, hormones out of whack … I have no patience. I am arguing with family members, pissed at people who aren't more sensitive to what I am going through.

Sophie, introduced earlier in the chapter, also felt disturbed about the apparent changes in her behaviour as she underwent fertility treatments, deeply concerned that she could not "control" herself. Like Patricia, she felt unable to manage her taken-for-granted everyday interactions as expressed in a journal entry:

> I hate it! This is not who I am nor who I want to be. I DO NOT bring my emotions to work, I DO NOT take my personal frustrations out on my co-workers, and I DO NOT treat my husband like I wish he would just go away. Apparently this is who I am now. I do all these things and more. It's horrible! I logically understand that my body is going through a lot with the drugs and hormones, so I should allow myself some changes. But then again I don't logically understand why I can't control myself. I don't know who I am, my employees are frightened of me, and my husband is worried about me. I am usually extremely helpful at work and people always feel that they can come to me with questions … but not anymore. I snip at them, tell them they'll have to figure it out, and basically tell them to eff off … I should be able to have a bit of restraint even when I don't want to … I'm done. Thanks for reading. Sorry you had to read. Please make me feel better by telling me you are all crazy too. :)

Opening her brief response with humour ("Welcome to insanity"), Brenda showed herself in tune with Sophie's self-mocking stance. She revealed similar difficulties in the past, noting intense anger towards others and her desire to "cut" them verbally, thus serving to normalise Sophie's behaviour. In the spirit of positive thinking, and implying that her own endeavours had culminated in success, Brenda encouraged her to continue the journey because it would be "worth it in the end".

In questioning the toll that the endless rounds of IF treatments were having on their lives, some of the women were driven to an existentially oriented search for meaning. Why had they been handed the card of infertility? What had they done to deserve it? Nowhere is the crisis of biographical disruption more clearly and poignantly illustrated than at these moments. In the aftermath of Patricia's third failed IVF attempt, we witness one such moment of crisis recorded in her journal, as she tries to make sense of her "IF journey" thus far:

> I am days away from my 42nd birthday and I just want to crawl into a hole! I don't want to look aging in the face anymore because I realise that is why I am having such a hard time getting pregnant. I don't know why it can't be easy for me like so many others. What did I do to deserve this fate? I waited 40 years to meet my soul mate and finally get married and now we are being denied a family of our own. We are not well off and probably can't afford to adopt (although we will look into it further). We love each other so much and instead of getting what we want IF is pushing us apart. The constant worrying, emotional turmoil, injections, doctor appointments, lack of intimacy and disappointment in the end is just destroying who I am ... who we are. None of it is fair! ...
>
> I want to be happy for all of the lovely women on here who are making their dreams come true, but it is so hard to read about their joy when I am suffering every day and feeling like a hamster on a wheel getting nowhere! I just don't think I can continue to read about BFP's (even though I am so glad they are happening ... both because they are deserved and because it proves that it DOES happen!). I think I need a hiatus.
>
> We are thinking of trying again ... I find myself doing nothing but writing about it, reading about it, researching it, worrying about it and it DEFINES me at this point. I want others to stop looking at me with sad eyes or telling me to stay positive because it's gonna happen! I just want to be ME ... the friend, co-worker, sister, daughter, wife that people like for who I am and not for what I am trying to achieve or what I am so sadly dealing with.

Imprisoned by the "constant worrying" and "emotional turmoil" of unre-
lenting rounds of failed IF treatments, which seem entirely to define her
selfhood, Patricia felt shut away from her hitherto taken-for-granted roles
of "friend", "co-worker", "sister" and "daughter". The experience of infertility had robbed her of the exercise and maintenance of these key social
bonds (Steuber and Solomon 2008, p. 839). "None of it is fair", she
exclaimed. Having "waited 40 years" to meet her "soul mate" and "finally
get married", only to be "denied a family" seemed incomprehensible. The
statement—"We love each other so much and instead of getting what we
want IF is pushing us apart"—captured her incredulity that such an outcome were possible when they had *all* the ingredients necessary for good
parenting: maturity, a loving relationship, employment, economic security,
and a strong desire to have children. On the face of it, their fate seemed
morally unjust, especially without an explanation to make sense of it. How
could she bring the messiness, the ambiguities and uncertainties of the
situation, into the "wholeness" of a "followable" story (Patterson 2002,
p. 77), through which to explain the situation to herself and to others? At
the same time, *how* could she relinquish the dream of having a family? This
predicament was excruciatingly painful, especially when one saw others'
"dreams come true", both online and in the offline environment. We
examine the key theme of "the pregnant other" in the next chapter, including the moral dimensions associated with the women's observations of
those they saw as undeserving of the "privilege" of motherhood.

Several months later, when consulting her RE, Patricia experienced
something of a turning point in recognising the extent to which their IF
struggle had taken over their lives. Not an entirely new insight for her,
however, it appeared to carry greater significance in this context because
it was introduced by the RE. In a lengthy journal entry, Patricia pondered
the matter in sorrowful contemplation:

> He took the time to be very caring with me and my DH and explain every-
> thing. While talking to him he said: 'I know that spending all of this time
> trying to get pregnant is very stressful and difficult and starts to define your
> whole relationship.' … When we left my DH turned to me and said, 'I
> don't even remember what our lives were like before we started all of this. I
> do remember though that we had a good social life and were happier peo-
> ple.' This is so true and made me so sad.

Patricia underlined very lucidly the emotional ramifications of the IF experience, and its ripple effects into their social networks:

> Our struggle has become all we talk about, think about, save money for, cry about and dream about. People don't know how to talk to us about anything else anymore or look at us without sympathy in their eyes. We hardly ever go anywhere or do anything fun.

Not only had social relations become fractured and awkward; the everyday labour involved in trying to have a baby "consumed" her physical energies and demanded a regime of self-discipline, exacting routines and calculations, obliterating their spontaneity:

> I'm exhausted all the time from the toll the stims take on me, as well as all of the running around to acupuncturists and early morning RE appointments, retrievals and transfers. We have NO SEX life anymore!! I am either exhausted, feeling fat and gross and in no mood when we can do it, or it's time for a retrieval and … we can't do anything … I realise that having a baby has consumed me and I no longer have an identity or enjoy day to day life. Everything is about counting days, seeing doctors, Googling signs, symptoms, stories, remedies, calling attorneys and social workers, figuring out where money will come from … STRESS, STRESS, STRESS.

Akin to a mini-ethnography of the lived experiences of infertility, Patricia evoked its damaging effects on self and other at the micro-social level, showing that infertility invades and turns one's world upside down, encroaching on and reshaping all manner of everyday routines (Steuber and Solomon 2008, p. 839). In their content analysis of blogs posted to several infertility-focused OSGs, Steuber and Solomon (2008, p. 840) reported that the problem of "instrumental" romance was frequently raised by participants: not only did IF eclipse people's lives, "it also contaminated romantic and sexual intimacy", as illustrated in Patricia's journal entry (see Chap. 6). She painted a stirring picture of an overwrought self, touching on the question of when, and how, to end the roller-coaster of "trying to conceive"? How much stress can (or should) one endure?

In concluding this section of the chapter, we weave together some of the key preoccupations voiced by women who had been "trying to conceive" for many years: the seeming futility of their efforts of working on the self, the thwarting of their dreams of motherhood, and questions of who they were and who they could be after the loss of those dreams. Edith's exchange with Mandy on the general discussion board exemplified the irrevocability of these losses (Jaffe 2017). Introducing herself, Edith explained that she and her DH had been "trying" for over twelve years; they achieved several pregnancies but none had advanced beyond two months. All she had ever wanted since childhood were "children of my own"; now she felt she wanted to "give up". Using a very haunting image, Edith described feeling as if she were being "mocked by nature", especially since she saw herself at odds with her "fertile" siblings, all of whom had children. In responding, Mandy noted a shared history in that she had been trying to conceive for 10 years. She had tried "anything and everything" from clean eating, herbs, and exercise to meditation and positive thinking, reading "constantly" in an effort to take "excellent care" of her mind and body and, after noting these painstaking efforts, she concluded abruptly: "I just don't know." Mandy seemed to have come to the end of road: but how can one reconcile the failure of these interventions with the intense desire to become a mother? Edith thanked Mandy for her reply, grateful that at least she understood her "pain", which affirmed she was not "alone" in it. She then posed a rhetorical question, infused with despair: "If I wasn't meant to be a mother, what am I doing here?" How can one get by with an "intense need" to parent, coupled with a long history of reproductive failure? There is no answer.

The sentiments expressed by Edith and Mandy were amongst the bleakest and despairing of the posts we examined, particularly because they seem to have come to the end of the road. After engaging in an array of labours to heighten their chances of a healthy pregnancy, there was little else that fellow-participants could suggest within the constraints of the narrative environment of "Stronger Together". An empathic connection, and recognition of the experience of suffering, was the most they could offer.

Such admissions by Edith that she felt "mocked by nature" and the question of what she could be—was "meant to be"—if she could not achieve motherhood pointed to profound experiences of alienation. Here it seemed that these women felt estranged from their human potential as mothers, disconnected from their species-being. Unable to engage their physical and mental energies in a productive project of mothering, they were bereft of a story to guide them into the future. However, these circumstances were not explored, nor made explicit in the online exchanges. As argued above, the narrative environment of Stronger Together did not encourage discussion of when to stop IF treatments and how to live a meaningful life in the wake of multiple failed treatments. Thus the existentially oriented quest of how to live in the absence of motherhood—how to let go of the dream—could not be confronted in this online space.

Conclusion

This chapter has examined the women's accounts of how they experienced and managed their emotions, bodies and selves as they engaged in various medical and non-medical strategies to enhance their chances of falling pregnant. In conceptualising the OSG as a very particular narrative environment (Gubrium and Holstein 2009), we demonstrated the dominant frameworks the women used to construct, reflect on, and intervene in their own and fellow-participants' stories. Along with an emphasis on "positive thinking" as the main currency of exchange, the women's discursive resources also included various individualised strategies of "working" on the self: an illustration of the reach of biopolitics into their everyday lives. In support of previous studies (e.g. Malik and Coulson 2010), we found that the overwhelming majority of posts and online interactions focused on issues of emotion management and the provision of empathy and support, and significantly fewer on questions and advice about medical procedures.

Close readings of selected online exchanges also revealed to us specific perspectives that could not be voiced in the online support group. Most notably, Patricia touched on the "dark side" of positive thinking, probing its hoax-like quality, an interpretation not taken up by other group members. Patricia was acutely aware of departing from the received script and, as discussed above, engaged in her own "repair" work (Gubrium 2005,

p. 526). Questions of how long one ought to keep "trying", especially after multiple IVF failures, were also discouraged: participants did not venture into suggestions of how one might conceptualise a meaningful life in the absence of motherhood. On this latter point, we speculated that the absence of culturally prescribed narratives (i.e. available discourses-in-practice) to guide one's life beyond a series of failed IVF attempts meant that these women were usually compelled to make sense of their experiences of biographical disruption in isolation from others. While such conditions as cancer, depression and grief have been explored through numerous memoirs and autobiographies—thus constituting distinct sub-genres of the illness experience—the same cannot be said of infertility. Very few personal accounts of failed IF treatment journeys are available in the public domain. Julia Leigh's (2016) recent memoir, *Avalanche*, is an exception. It offers a discursive space for public narratives of self-identity and everyday life in the wake of failed IF treatments, and (public) recognition of the very particular forms of social suffering entailed in these experiences (see ABC TV 2016; Wilkinson and Kleinman 2016). We might therefore understand the participants of Stronger Together through their attempts to rework their "selves" in the particular narrative environment of the OSG, and in the broader context of the cultural logics of neoliberalism, therapy culture, and biomedical advances and constraints.

References

Australian Broadcasting Commission ABC TV. (2016). The Baby Business. *Four Corners* (Broadcast May-30). Retrieved from http://www.abc.net.au/4corners/stories/2016/05/30/4469652.htm.

Barak, A., Boniel-Nissim, M., & Suler, J. (2008). Fostering Empowerment in Online Support Groups. *Computers in Human Behavior, 24*(5), 1867–1883.

Beck, U. (1992). *Risk Society: Towards a New Modernity*. Newbury Park: Sage.

Beck, U., & Beck-Gernsheim, E. (2002). *Individualization: Institutionalized Individualism and Its Social and Political Consequences*. London; Thousand Oaks, CA: Sage.

Broom, A. (2009). Intuition, Subjectivity and Le bricoleur: Cancer Patients' Accounts of Negotiating a Plurality of Therapeutic Options. *Qualitative Health Research, 19*(8), 1050–1059.

Broom, A., & Tovey, P. (2007). Therapeutic Pluralism? Evidence, Power and Legitimacy in UK Cancer Services. *Sociology of Health & Illness, 29*(3), 551–569.

Bruner, J. (1987). Life as Narrative. *Social Research, 54*(1), 11–32.

Bury, M. (1982). Chronic Illness as Biographical Disruption. *Sociology of Health & Illness, 4*(2), 167–182.

Crawshaw, P. (2012). Governing at a Distance: Social Marketing and the Bio(Politics) of Responsibility. *Social Science & Medicine, 75,* 200–2007.

Didion, J. (2005). *The Year of Magical Thinking.* New York: Knopf.

Doka, K. J. (1989). *Disenfranchised Grief: Recognizing Hidden Sorrow.* Lexington: Lexington Books.

Doka, K. J. (2002). *Disenfranchised Grief: New Directions, Challenges and Strategies for Practice.* Champaign, IL: Research Press.

Ettore, E. (2002). A Critical Look at the New Genetics: Conceptualizing the Links Between Reproduction, Gender and Bodies. *Critical Public Health, 12*(3), 237–250.

Francis, L. A. (1997). Ideology and Interpersonal Emotion Management: Redefining Identity in Two Support Groups. *Social Psychology Quarterly, 60*(2), 153–171.

Frank, A. (2010). *Letting Stories Breathe: A Socio-Narratology.* Chicago: University of Chicago Press.

Giddens, A. (1991). *Modernity and Self-Identity: Self and Society in the Late Modern Age.* Cambridge: Polity.

Gubrium, J. F. (2005). Introduction: Narrative Environments and Social Problems. *Social Problems, 52*(4), 525–528.

Gubrium, J. F., & Holstein, J. A. (2000). The Self in a World of Going Concerns. *Symbolic Interaction, 23*(2), 95–115.

Gubrium, J. F., & Holstein, J. A. (2009). *Analyzing Narrative Reality.* Thousand Oaks, CA: Sage.

Hinton, L., Kurinczuk, J. J., & Ziebland, S. (2010). Infertility; Isolation and the Internet: A Qualitative Interview Study. *Patient Education and Counseling, 81*(3), 436–441.

Hitchens, C. (2012). *Mortality.* London: Atlantic Books.

Hochschild, A. R. (1979). Emotion Work, Feeling Rules, and Social Structure. *American Journal of Sociology, 85*(3), 551–575.

Holstein, J. A., & Gubrium, J. F. (2000). *The Self We Live By: Narrative Identity in a Postmodern World.* New York: Oxford University Press.

Illouz, E. (2003). *Oprah Winfrey and the Glamour of Misery.* New York: Columbia University Press.

Illouz, E. (2008). *Saving the Modern Soul: Therapy, Emotions, and the Culture of Self-Help*. Berkeley, CA: University of California Press.

Jaffe, J. (2017). Reproductive Trauma: Psychotherapy for Pregnancy Loss and Infertility Clients from a Reproductive Story Perspective. *Psychotherapy, 54*(4), 380–385.

Jasper, J. M. (2014). Constructing Indignation: Anger Dynamics in Protest Movements. *Emotion Review, 6*(3), 208–213.

Leigh, J. (2016). *Avalanche: A Love Story*. Melbourne: Penguin Group Australia.

Lewis, C. S. (1961). *A Grief Observed*. London: Faber.

Lourde, A. (1980). *The Cancer Journals*. San Francisco: Aunt Lute Books.

Lupton, D. (2012). 'Precious Cargo': Foetal Subjects, Risk and Reproductive Citizenship. *Critical Public Health, 22*(3), 329–340.

Lupton, D. (2013). *Risk*. London; New York: Routledge.

Malik, S. H., & Coulson, N. S. (2010). Coping with Infertility Online: An Examination of Self-Help Mechanisms in an Online Infertility Support Group. *Patient Education and Counseling, 81*(2), 315–318.

May, V. (2012). Narrative Analysis and Interpretive Phenomenological Analysis. In C. Seale (Ed.), *Researching Society and Culture* (pp. 441–458). *London: Sage.*

Patterson, W. (2002). Narrative Imaginings: The Liminal Zone in Narratives of Trauma. In W. Patterson (Ed.), *Strategic Narrative: New Perspectives on the Power of Personal and Cultural Stories* (pp. 71–88). Lanham, MD: Lexington Books.

Petersen, A. (1996). Risk and the Regulated Self: The Discourse of Health Promotion as Politics of Uncertainty. *Australia and New Zealand Journal of Sociology, 31*(1), 44–57.

Richardson, L. (1990). Narrative and Sociology. *Journal of Contemporary Ethnography, 19*(1), 116–135.

Ricoeur, P. (1991). Life in Quest of Narrative (trans. D. Wood). In D. Wood (Ed.), *On Paul Ricoeur: Narrative and Interpretation* (pp. 20–33). London: Routledge.

Saleebey, D. (1994). Culture, Theory, and Narrative: The Intersections of Meaning in Practice. *Social Work, 39*(4), 351–359.

Silva, J. (2013). *Coming Up Short: Working-Class Adulthood in an Age of Uncertainty*. New York: Oxford University Press.

Singleton, A., Abeles, P., & Smith, I. C. (2016). Online Social Networking and Psychological Experiences: The Perceptions of Young People with Mental Health Difficulties. *Computers in Human Behavior, 61*(August), 394–403.

Steuber, K. R., & Solomon, D. H. (2008). Relational Uncertainty, Partner Interference, and Infertility: A Qualitative Study of Discourse within Online Forums. *Journal of Social and Personal Relationships, 25*(5), 831–855.

Styron, W. (1990). *Darkness Visible: A Memoir of Madness*. New York: Random House.

White, M., & Dorman, S. M. (2001). Receiving Social Support Online: Implications for Health Education. *Health Education Research, 16*(6), 693–707.

Wilkinson, I., & Kleinman, A. (2016). *A Passion for Society: How We Think About Human Suffering*. Oakland, CA: University of California Press.

Wurtzel, E. (1994). *Prozac Nation: Young and Depressed in America*. Boston: Houghton Mifflin.

5

Relationships in a Fertile World: Negotiating Alliances and the "Pregnant Other"

Anne-Maree Sawyer

"This journey is such a tough one and only someone who has experienced it can know how deeply it affects you." (Stronger Together participant)
"I had three friends announce they were pregnant within 2 weeks of each other … It feels almost like a personal attack!" (Stronger Together participant)

Introduction

This chapter examines the destabilisation of key relationships in the women's lives in the context of their experiences of infertility. Specifically, we focus on how these experiences affected their interactions with family, friends and work colleagues. (The women's accounts of their relationships with their spouses are explored in Chap. 6.) The Stronger Together site offered the women a secure place to "vent" about their interactions with

A.-M. Sawyer (✉)
La Trobe University, Melbourne, Australia
e-mail: a.sawyer@latrobe.edu.au

© The Author(s) 2019
P. Billett, A.-M. Sawyer, *Infertility and Intimacy in an Online Community*,
Palgrave Macmillan Studies in Family and Intimate Life,
https://doi.org/10.1057/978-1-137-44981-8_5

significant others—the pain and indignation of confronting others' seemingly unfeeling reactions; whether or not to disclose their struggles with infertility; how to deal with the news of other women's pregnancies; and how to regard the infertility "advice" proffered by relatives and close friends.

Women frequently used the site to seek feedback on their own emotional reactions, as demonstrated in Serena's post to the general discussion board. She was concerned over a particular friendship. Her best friend had been "hanging out constantly" with another woman, who had recently announced her pregnancy in public "with no sensitivity" towards Serena's feelings. Both the other woman and her best friend were expecting babies, and were therefore part of the "mommy club", and Serena felt "jealous" and "betrayed" at being left out of their social get-togethers. In her post, she sought advice on what to do, how to regulate her feelings; she felt she should do or say "something" because she was due to start "team teaching" with her best friend in a week or so and did not want to go into this situation with "hurt feelings". At the same time, Serena acknowledged that it was very likely that her best friend had "no idea" of the hurt she had caused and the last thing she wanted to do was cause a "drama" in their relationship or behave like a "jealous high schooler".

Several different threads of pain were encapsulated in Serena's post, all of them commonly voiced by other participants on the site: the insensitivity of fertile others when announcing their pregnancies; the feeling of being "left out", "literally" and figuratively; puzzling over how to contain feelings of jealousy and resentment; and whether, and how, to confront others about the far-reaching effects of their behaviours on the self. Applying a micro-sociological lens to her sense-making process raises the question of the extent to which fertile others *are* able to "take the role" of those who are infertile. As David Karp (2001, p. 86) so eloquently explained in his study of family care-givers of people with severe mental illnesses, "To genuinely care for another person presumes efforts to empathize with them, to feel what they feel, to try to see the world from their standpoint, to 'take their role.' Of course, all role-taking is approximate since we can never fully understand what another person is experiencing." A relationship with a best friend carries an expectation that the two people involved will make a concerted effort to understand the other's particular circumstances, to empathise and make adjustments accordingly. Yet for such a stigmatised and poorly understood condition as infertility, it is genuinely difficult for a "healthy" fertile individual to empathise with a person suffering from infertility. Without the emotional knowledge of how infertility actually feels, the fertile other is hard-pressed to imagine how injurious her behaviour and apparent lack of consideration might feel to the person on the receiving end of it. While Serena attempts to "take the role" of her best friend, imagining that she did not—or could not—realise the "hurt" she had caused, she also touched on a further thread of experience, often voiced tacitly by others on the site: to what extent is it legitimate to feel injured, in the first place? This is captured in her fear that, should she confront her friend about the "hurt" she inflicted, she risks being seen as a "drama" queen or a "jealous high schooler". The crux of many such ponderings involved a complex criss-crossing of imagining and puzzling over the motivations behind the other person's behaviours and one's own reactions. Producing a form of emotional entrapment, these ponderings pleaded for emotional regulation and emotional justice. And it is this quality of entrapment that seemed to define and impel the *destabilisation* of the women's key (offline) relationships that we examine in this chapter.

Thus the central question framing this chapter is: How did the women construct, negotiate, and manage their emotions (Hochschild 1979; Lively and Weed 2014) in relationships with significant others? What kind of definitional work did they utilise? Through examining a range of online posts and journal entries we can see that the OSG offered the women a safe place to "second guess" the motives and reactions of others and of themselves; we often witness the women "thinking out loud" as they try to make sense of their emotional reactions. In this chapter, we also continue our emerging observations concerning the "triangulation" of the women's key relationships and intimacies. (See Chaps. 3 and 6 for further discussion.) This reflects a particular pattern in the way the women perceived themselves through their actual and imagined interactions with family, friends and work colleagues; their partners; and, their online relationships. These three intersecting reference points seemed to provide material for self-construction, self-validation and self-regulation, and for a re-grouping of their key intimacies. Significantly, the women frequently saw their online relationships as providing a depth of "recognition" (Frost 2016) and empathy far beyond the support offered by those without lived experience of infertility. The following two excerpts demonstrate the depth of the recognition sought and received by participants in the online space (Barak et al. 2008).

The first concerns a post to the general discussion board made by Ellen, who felt distressed and alone after learning that a good friend had given birth earlier in the day. She opened her post by saying she was "back" on the discussion board because, although feeling "super happy" for her friend, it was "still" difficult to hear this news. She had phoned to tell her mother, and the "excitement" she expressed was a sad "reminder" to Ellen that she was not the source of her mother's joy. To Ellen, her mother's excitement felt like a "kick": an invitation to "imagine" how much happier she would sound if, instead, it were the birth of Ellen's child. Ellen acknowledged that these thoughts were simply in her "head", yet also inevitable: "just the way it is". Realising her husband would not appreciate her reading of the telephone call to her mother, she had decided to post to the general discussion board since it was very likely she would "find someone on here" who did understand; and if not, she could at least give "vent" to her feelings.

The triangular patterning is evident here: Ellen's consciousness of her mother's reaction; her doubts that her husband would understand; and her need to "find someone on here" to recognise her inner turmoil. She assessed herself, in the main, from her mother's standpoint, giving voice to the shame and sadness she felt in failing to deliver news of her own child's birth. (Here we might also recall Bernadette's post anticipating the "shame spiral" that would engulf her if fertility treatments proved unsuccessful; see Chap. 4.) Shame is often referred to as one of the "self-conscious" or "moral" emotions, along with pride, guilt, and embarrassment, because it points to the evaluative cultural norms that tell us what is right or wrong, good or bad, acceptable or unacceptable (Harkness and Hinton 2014, p. 451). According to Chase and Walker (2012, pp. 739–40), shame "entails a negative assessment of the self made with reference to one's own aspirations and the perceived expectations of others, and is manifested as a sense of powerlessness and feeling small". Whereas shame concerns negative self-evaluations over which a person has very limited control, guilt refers to "an internal negative assessment of certain behaviour which … could have been avoided" (Chase and Walker 2012, p. 743). In everyday parlance, guilt and shame are often used interchangeably. However, we argue that shame, rather than guilt, charac-terised the entrapment and destabilisation the women experienced in their relationships with their partners, family members, friends and work colleagues in the context of their struggles with infertility. Ellen's imagined "kick" from her mother for not having fulfilled her maternal aspirations reflects her "sense of powerlessness and feeling small" (Chase and Walker 2012, p. 743), a punitive judgement of self as "bad" and "unacceptable".

In the second excerpt, Elisabeth sought succour and self-validation from the OSG following her first failed IUI. In a journal post, she explained how she awoke in the middle of the night to "an overwhelming sadness", and tried to distract herself with the television and internet:

> My husband woke up and I told him I couldn't stop crying, that I was too sad. He told me to let him know if I needed anything and then fell right back asleep. Feeling very isolated. Now I'm just sitting here and bawling like an idiot. I hate this.

Lydia responded to Elisabeth's journal post, disclosing that she had suf-fered a "mini breakdown" not long after her first failed IUI. She described having been very angry and upset, admitting that all she could do "was cry". Lydia assured Elisabeth that her emotions were "normal", and the IF "journey" was so "tough" that only those who had experienced it first hand could "know how deeply it affects you". She noted that she felt exactly the "same way" as Elisabeth. Lydia advised her to "stay focused on the positives"—to hold onto the conviction that "it WILL happen" by keeping the ultimate goal at the forefront of her mind. This very empathic response seemed to comfort Elisabeth. It offered her a modicum of hope, and a means of re-framing and managing her emotions, as attested by the update she posted several hours later:

> Didn't get much sleep, but feeling better this morning. I'm going to try to keep my mind occupied and tell myself it's okay to take a day to kind of do nothing and try to relax ...
>
> I know I'll feel better in a week or so when we start a new cycle. It always feels good to be making progress towards a pregnancy ... I'm going to try to focus on the positive, and the fact that I can relax and not worry if every little twinge is some kind of sign.

An element of "triangulation" is also evident in this encounter. "Feeling very isolated", Elisabeth felt pushed to seek solace online after her husband "fell right back asleep", a move that possibly helped to destabilise her relationship with him. Lydia's assertion that "only someone" with firsthand experience of IF could know the grief it caused contributed to their shared intimacy. It also facilitated Elisabeth's experience of this online support as productive and authentic: "authentic" in terms of the genuineness of Lydia's understanding, her lived experience of the emotions associated with failed infertility treatments, and hence the legitimacy of the advice proffered. We can therefore surmise that such online encounters potentially engendered a re-grouping of the women's key intimacies and alliances in the context of their experiences of infertility, with their online relationships taking centre-stage while significant others (partners; family, friends, work colleagues) were relegated to the sidelines.

This chapter is organised into three main sections. First, we examine the women's accounts of how they negotiated relationships with their families, particularly their mothers since many were concerned about their failure to provide grandchildren. Secondly, we discuss their accounts of relationships with friends and colleagues; and finally, we discuss the women's observations of "undeserving" pregnant others. Hearing the news of another woman's pregnancy was often met with intense anguish. A reminder of their own failure to conceive, these events aroused a range of conflicted emotions—overwhelming sadness, the shame of not achieving motherhood, jealousy, betrayal, anger, and guilt over their inability to share in the other's joy. The force of these emotional responses often surprised the women themselves. Some felt swallowed up by their emotions, overwhelmed at not being the person they thought they were or wanted to be, especially if the pregnant other were a close friend or family member. Others felt plunged into a mire of unpredictable and undesirable reactions—punished by the news of another women's joy, more particularly if her path to pregnancy had been short and trouble-free. As Elisabeth declared in her online journal: "I really feel like the universe is just rubbing it in. It's so hard to keep hearing about people in my age group getting pregnant left and right."

Family Relationships

Mothers

The women's accounts of their interactions with their mothers frequently involved anger and frustration, and unfulfilled expectations of unconditional support and empathy. These encounters were often riven with intense disappointment that their mother had not taken their part; that she had not "displayed" (Dermott and Seymour 2011) a wellspring of maternal beneficence and succour. In some cases, the women took issue with their mothers' reactions to their infertility—the particular attitudes and the "advice" offered. It must be said, however, that women who experienced conflict with their mothers were more likely to post about it on the general discussion board and in their online journals, compared with those who felt well supported. Given that Stronger Together is oriented to "venting" and (emotional) problem-solving, women experiencing conflict with their mothers were likely to be over-represented in this online space. (Moreover, as noted in the introduction, the focus of this book is on the issues and problems raised on the Stronger Together site; for this reason we have approached this OSG as a very particular narrative environment.)

Joan, who made lengthy entries in her online journal, described a very painful and troubling encounter with her mother. She had been trying to conceive for several years, and was also struggling with over-weight and depression and with the ongoing side-effects of IVF treatments. At the same time, Joan and her husband were finding it difficult to manage their day-to-day bills. While recognising that her mother meant "well", Joan felt "angry and hurt" by her conviction that people choose how to react to life's problems:

Ok, I know my mum means well when she tries to 'encourage' me about all of this [IF-related issues], but I can't help feeling angry and hurt by what she says. To her, most 'negative' things are a choice, including depression. According to her, you can CHOOSE to sit there and wallow and feel bad for no reason OR you can CHOOSE to get off the couch/out of bed and be happy about life.

It's obvious to me that she's never been truly depressed in life. Yes, she's had a rough life and all, but seriously, if she truly suffered from depression she'd know you can't choose that crap, you can't choose to just be happy when everything in you is screaming pain and sadness!

Joan was also infuriated by the nature of the "advice" her mother offered, not only because her mother was a "registered nurse" and "should" have known better, but because it only echoed what she and her husband had already considered:

Oh, and she's a registered nurse on top of that, so she SHOULD know that depression is now classified as a mental illness and is NOT chosen, but I digress …

Normally her advice about things is ridiculous to me, so I rarely if ever talk to her about things. I mentioned something in passing today because it had relevance to something funny that happened. Her instant reaction to the comment of my hubby being sad/depressed about the IF and everyone at work having kids or announcing pregnancies was to immediately try to 'diagnose' problems and tell me how my hubby's recent finding of a major UI [urinary infection] causing bladder issues and inflammation (of the bladder and upper urethra) could be causing "extra" troubles with our IF struggles. Like we hadn't thought of that ourselves?

Joan acknowledged that her mother did make an effort to be "helpful" but her reactions and suggestions were "not helping". She was angry because, as she reported, her mother seemed unable to cease her "unhelpful advice"—and this fuelled the negative dynamics between them. Nevertheless, Joan conceded that her mother had not pressed her to provide grandchildren as frequently as in the past. Yet, she felt "guilty" over the anger she harboured towards her mother, akin to a form of emotional entrapment, and was uncertain of how to deal with it: "I don't know what to say to her to get her to see that her opinions on my IF hurt more than they help." Still, like many of the other women, Joan questioned her reading of this very troubling emotional situation, emphasising that:

I hate how IF makes every day a struggle and how *even small comments send me into a spiral of anger, pain and sadness*. I hate that I'm crying right now because of all of this. (Italics added)

As in Serena's post that opened this chapter, Joan wondered if she might be over-reacting to her mother's suggestions, because "even small comments" sent her into "a spiral of anger, pain and sadness". She was concerned that her seemingly heightened sensitivity might be the cause of the problems in their relationship. Again, we see an example of a Stronger Together participant puzzling over her emotions in an effort to regulate them and attain emotional justice. At the heart of Joan's "struggle" are the questions: Do I have a legitimate emotional claim? Are my emotions defensible?

Mothers' Day

Not surprisingly, Mothers' Day was imbued with heightened anguish for many of the women, a tormenting reminder of the loss of their dreams of motherhood. Some women described feeling wounded afresh when the Day was discussed and anticipated by family and friends. Others felt troubled by the pressure to contain their own sadness while displaying happiness and voicing good wishes to the mothers in their midst. In the early stages of the IF journey, relations with their own mothers could be tense and awkward in the context of family events associated with Mothers' Day. However, in some situations, especially after several years of languishing in "IF limbo", their mother might have learned to "avoid" stress-inducing conversations about Mothers' Day, as shown in one of Joan's journal entries:

> My Mum's thankfully not making that big a deal of Mother's Day this year. I think it finally got through to her that it hurts me when she goes on and on about it. She was dropping hints about what she'd like, which for once is not a TV series or something stupidly expensive. She wants garden decor items, which can be expensive, but I know a few places I can get a few items for cheaper. I think I may just get her a gift card to somewhere and get her to pick out her own garden items. She'll be pissy with that, but hey, at least she can choose something she likes.

A few days later, she reflected on the Day, which had been a source of great distress in the past. Now "even" her friends "avoided the topic, too".

One senses that Joan feels respected, that these significant others have been "nice" to her in adjusting their behaviours, in taking the role of the other:

> Also, yesterday was an ok day for me. I talked to my mum for a little bit, and other than saying 'Happy Mother's Day' and talking about the gift she wanted from me and telling me the names of the plants she got from my brothers, we didn't talk about the day. We pretty much ignored the fact that it was Mother's Day. DH called his mum and talked to her for a bit, more playing catch up than anything else … My friends even avoided the topic too, which was nice.

Because the prospect of Mothers' Day often triggered feelings of loss and despair, other people's so-called normal approaches to marking the Day were seen as newly problematic by the women. They found themselves in situations that called for intense emotion management and self-analysis, frequently ruminating over their own reactions and concerned about their readings of others' behaviours. Stronger Together participants often felt deeply conflicted in terms of how they dealt with the Day, as exemplified in an exchange between Janet and Lottie. Posting to the general discussion board, Janet asked if others were "struggling" with Mothers' Day. She admitted to having a "really hard time" this year, having just received news of her second failed IVF cycle. She felt she was "still mourning" and therefore did not want to celebrate the Day with her brothers and their children: "I … just can't do it." As a result she felt "selfish" because her mother had been "such a great support" during her IVF cycles; she saw her lack of enthusiasm for the Day as a slight against her mother, and felt burdened by a sense of disquiet she could not resolve.

Responding to Janet's post, Lottie described her own very conflicted and painful experience of Mothers' Day as a consequence of her sister's insensitive behaviour when announcing her pregnancy. Lottie had confided in her sister as one of the "few" who knew the details of her "struggle" with infertility; she now regretted having done so. For some weeks, Lottie had suspected her sister was "pregnant again" from various signs she observed, but nothing was said on the matter. Assuming she might be waiting until Mothers' Day to make the announcement, Lottie had prepared to protect herself by sending a letter to her sister, along with a short magazine article relating "how hard" Mothers' Day could be for women "struggling with infertility". On the Saturday before Mother's Day the extended family met at Lottie's grandmother's house and her sister announced her pregnancy then. Consequently, Lottie had a "big argument" with her sister, who asked why she was so "upset". Lottie tried to explain, but with little effect. Her sister repeated her announcement at their other grandmother's house on the Sunday (Mother's Day). "It was the worst" experience, Lottie exclaimed in her post. Late on Mothers' Day she sent a text message to her sister, expressing disappointment in the way the announcements had been made. Lottie found her sister's response "very selfish" and dismissive, and felt she could no longer rely on her as a chief support.

Multiple hurts are embedded in Lottie's story. From the first signs of pregnancy, she felt shut out of her sister's personal world, particularly in light of their history of shared intimacies. Her sister's two pregnancy announcements over the Mother's Day weekend intensified Lottie's suffering; she could not understand why her sister had apparently not taken her feelings into consideration when she was aware of them. And, at the end of the weekend, Lottie tried to reach out to her sister, to explain why she was "upset"—only to feel "dismissed". Like many other accounts of painful interactions with a significant other over their announcement of a pregnancy, Lottie's experience called for emotional regulation and emotional justice. She was left to deal with the emotional fall-out from the encounter with her sister. Lottie had expected a semblance of compassion from her sister in exchange for revealing how "upset" she had been by the pregnancy announcements, having paved the way earlier with the magazine article. Candace Clark's (1997) pioneering work on the micro-politics of emotional exchange is useful in thinking through this encounter. Of the three exchange logics identified by Clark, the principle of complementary role requirements seems most applicable: the expectation that "people should give to others because their social roles oblige them to do so" (Clark 1997, p. 134). According to this logic, a sister *should* provide understanding and support as a consequence of the close family connection. Instead, Lottie felt "dismissed", silenced—under-compensated in this asymmetrical exchange—and left to manage her emotions in isolation. The norm of unconditional family love and support had not been realised, and she was forced to bear the burden of resolving this painful encounter. Time and again, such disquieting and destabilising encounters with family members, friends, and work colleagues were experienced as an assault on the self. These posts demonstrated a reaching out to online others for the recognition and empathy not available from significant others in their offline worlds, which generated a re-grouping of the women's key intimacies.

Pregnant Others Amongst Friends and Colleagues

Dealing with the "pregnant other" was a key theme in the women's posts, as noted above. Learning about others' success in conceiving was frequently a source of great distress, especially when this news came unexpectedly. Women often sought support from their online "friends" to debrief about the shock of the news, and to get a handle on their emotional reactions—Were they over-reacting? How could they make sense of what had happened? Many posts appealed for emotional regulation and emotional justice: the drive to understand and disentangle their own reactions from those of others, and to rein in their seemingly runaway emotions that defied control.

In a journal entry titled "Other people's happiness", Elisabeth offered a very reflective account of her conflicted reaction to the news of two pregnancies:

> There's been two people who've had babies in the last couple of weeks, one my husband's cousin, one an old friend. (The cousin is especially tough on me, because she and her husband got married just over a year ago, and I found out she was pregnant when we visited his family, and there she was, 8 months pregnant. I had to hold it together while I looked at the ultrasounds. I still have an irrational anger at my husband for not knowing she was pregnant. It was really awful to have it sprung on me.) I really should just block everyone who has small children. I can't handle seeing

the pictures without bawling, but I look anyway. I feel horrible that I just can't be happy for them without feeling so sad for myself ...
A couple of days ago I watched a video that another friend posted for her toddler and infant. It was so sweet, but then I had to get up and go cry in the bathroom where my husband couldn't see me. I'm so tired of feeling sorry for myself, especially when there is so much that is good in my life, but part of me really can't help it. The tears come even when I try so hard to stop them. I'm just so happy that none of my really close friends are even close to TTC, so as bad as it makes me feel, I just need to put everyone else on hold and just focus on them. That's not wrong, is it?

Again, we see the complex and tricky process of emotion management (Hochschild 1979; Lively and Weed 2014) with Elisabeth oscillating between suppressing her anguish ("I had to hold it together while I looked at the ultrasounds"), and failing to do so ("The tears come even when I try so hard to stop them"). A manifestation of the triangulation process is also evident in the "irrational anger" she felt towards her husband for not knowing his cousin was pregnant, and the need to "go cry in the bathroom" away from him after viewing the video of her friend's children—and afterwards in revealing her innermost feelings in the online space. Her act of posting to Stronger Together seemed to provide a means of "working through", a form of problem-solving, because it generated the realisation that perhaps she needed to "put everyone else on hold" and just attend to her "really close" friends who were "not TTC" (Pennebaker and Evans 2014; Pennebaker and Smyth 2016).

There was a strong moral aspect to Elisabeth's revelations, as demonstrated in similar accounts in the online space. She felt "bad" about feeling "happy" that none of her "really close friends" were "even close to TTC", thus questioning the legitimacy of her feelings. This was a significant defining feature of the experience of entrapment identified in the introduction to this chapter. Without culturally prescribed guides and narratives to frame these experiences, the women often felt cast adrift in a sea of uncertainty, bereft of meaning-making resources to make sense of their sharply conflicted feelings. We see this uncertainty expressed in Elisabeth's seeking after advice and reassurance in asking: "That's not wrong, is it?"

Some months later, Elisabeth decided to take a "break" from the IF treatments. All had been going well; she had lost some weight and had been painting the inside of the house as a longed-for change of focus. However, things began to unravel when her husband's ex-girlfriend added him as a "friend" on Facebook:

> I made a comment to the effect of, 'Oh great, she probably added you because she's pregnant.' I was sort of basing this on the past, when she found him out on MySpace around the time she got engaged.
>
> So we're … watching TV, and my husband's on his laptop, and he goes, 'You were right.' The bitch is pregnant! And I know that's why she chose now to find him. I really don't think she knows that we are going through IF, but I'm still pissed and sad and so, so bitter.
>
> I held it together for about five minutes; then I went upstairs and hid in our closet with all the lights off and cried my eyes out. My husband eventually went up to check on me, just when I was pulling it together. He tries. I appreciate that he tries. *But sometimes men just don't understand that all you want to do is cry and cry and let the pain bleed out of you.* I told him that as much as I appreciate the sentiment, I don't want to hear anything that begins with 'Think of it this way …' when I'm in that state. I don't want to think of it any way. I hate that I'm thinking of it at all.
>
> Whatever. I'll probably feel better tomorrow. I just needed to vent a little! (Italics added)

This excerpt shows very poignantly Elisabeth's struggle to manage her emotions, and the recognition that sometimes a visceral emotional release ("to cry and cry and let the pain bleed out of you") is necessary to expel some of the pain. The image of letting the pain "bleed out of you" is very affecting, suggesting a slow, tortured, and debilitating release. Perhaps, too, it indicates the inadequacy of words to convey such depth of despair, but also the potential for words to deepen the pain ("I hate that I'm thinking of it at all"). Yet again, we see the process of triangulation, with Elisabeth's husband pushed aside in preference for the online others with whom she can genuinely "vent".

Fast on the heels of the news of her husband's ex-girlfriend's pregnancy, Elisabeth faced another similar episode:

Randomly, some girl I went to high school with who I'm friends with on Facebook ... wrote that she is pregnant. Another one! At this point I really feel like the universe is just rubbing it in. It's so hard to keep hearing about people in my age group getting pregnant left and right. I blocked her like I've blocked everyone else who is pregnant or has just had a baby. Just can't deal with it right now.

   I don't want to be bitter. I want this struggle to be a test that I pass, one that makes me stronger in the long run. It's just hard to see the months, the years pass by and not feel like I'm any closer to my goal. I felt better after I told my husband I was sad. Holding it in was making it fester, so I'm glad I bled it out before it turned into something nasty. Writing it helps, too. Now, to sleep it off.

Elisabeth's representation of her psychic pain as an inflammatory condition conveys both the nature of her suffering, as deep-seated and visceral, and the means of relieving it ("Holding it in was making it fester, so I'm glad I bled it out before it turned into something nasty"). Here she touches on some key assumptions concerning the therapeutic ethos of self: the responsibility of individuals to identify their psychic pain, give voice to it in conversation with others and, finally, to overcome it (Illouz 2003, 2007). She "bleeds" it "out"—works through her pain—by talking to her husband. As Silva (2013, p. 167) explains:

> The therapeutic ethos has become *the* language for talking about the self. In this way, a new form of popular theodicy has taken root, one that views all suffering as purposeful and controllable: if we can only learn to manage our emotions, and thereby create a new relationship with our pasts, we can alleviate suffering and reach our true potential. (Illouz 2008) (Italics included)

Elisabeth yearned to know that her suffering had not been in vain: "I don't want to be bitter. I want this struggle to be a test that I pass, one that makes me stronger in the long run." These expressed needs reveal her personal efforts at self-regulation, together with the broader cultural expectation that individuals have the capacity to triumph over sadness and to grow emotionally "stronger" by "managing" their own suffering (Silva 2013, p. 19).

In response, Tayla identified with Elisabeth's plight and offered gentle guidance that reinforced the tenets of therapeutic selfhood and positive thinking. She noted that she, too, hated the "bitter feeling" Elisabeth had articulated. In an effort to help Elisabeth rethink her situation and suffering (Barak et al. 2008, p. 1876), Tayla argued that "everyone has a struggle in life": while *they* struggled with infertility, people "building their families" with apparent ease had very different troubles to bear, even if outsiders were oblivious to their particular trials and tribulations. To exemplify such hidden struggles, Tayla mentioned a man she had been nursing, who had only a week to live. Engaging in interpersonal emotion management, she encouraged Elisabeth to think more positively about her own struggles and the (projected) legacy of greater strength born out of suffering, asserting that she would "come out a stronger person in the end".

Not surprisingly, given the anguish of learning of others' pregnancies, the stress of managing "baby showers" was also much discussed amongst Stronger Together participants. In a post to the general discussion board, Helen explained that she and her partner had been forced to put their fertility treatments "on hold" for three years following a "horrible car accident". Very recently, they had "restarted" the process. Reflecting on the strains of the past few years, and the arduous treatments ahead of them, Helen now felt irritated and downhearted in finding herself "surrounded" by six pregnancies among "close" friends and family, all of who were due within four months of one another. "Dreading" the "upcoming months" with "all these showers", she hoped to find support from the online group—specifically, to deal with the "horrible", conflicted emotions she harboured concerning the pregnancies. Instead of feeling "happy and supportive", she was miserable and forlorn: "all I do is cry or kick into a day of depression". Her reaction constitutes a significant transgression from the feeling rules associated with receiving news of a pregnancy (Hochschild 1979), thus illustrating an experience of emotional entrapment.

Hana, Helen's first respondent, established an empathic connection early in her post, with a declaration of intimate support ("sending you hugs and strength"), and disclosure of her own experience as a "crappy friend". She then attempted to explain their unwelcome reactions to the news of significant others' pregnancies, noting that it was "very hard" to feel genuine happiness for others when "struggling for that same thing". Despite venturing into this definitional work, she could not convince herself that their reactions were "normal or expected or allowed". She tried to pull herself into the normative range of behaviours by stating that "of course" she felt "happy" for her friends who had children, and did not want them to struggle as she had, yet "sometimes" she failed to be "100% happy" about their news.

Even though Hana's suggestions were not very helpful in addressing her problem, Helen seemed to appreciate her empathy, posting that she "completely" understood her perspective. In her reply, Helen described herself as "very selfish" in relation to the pregnancies, with no clear pathway in view to regulate or rethink these emotions. As suggested in the previous chapter, there are no clear cultural guides for understanding and dealing with these (transgressive) feelings. Helen explained that the shock of hearing about the pregnancies was all the more "difficult" because none of the women had struggled to conceive: none were planned pregnancies and several were onto their second or third pregnancies, thus widening the gap between her childlessness and their experiences of parenthood. As sociologists and social scientists have noted, an experience of "normal ageing" depends on undergoing major life-course transitions in the correct sequence and at the "appropriate" age, notwithstanding variations in age-related norms associated with social class and historical location (Hunt 2017; Karp 2001, p. 142). Helen, along with the many others whose voices we hear in this book, expressed the pain of being "off time" or "left behind", an experience that seemed to deepen with the passing of time. She reasoned that the "older" she got, the "more difficult" it became, noting that the news of births in earlier years had not elicited such distress.

In contrast with Hana's ambivalent stance, Sigrid was very forthright in her response, arguing to normalise their "horrible" feelings concerning others' pregnancies. She admitted to "deleting" anyone who was pregnant, or had a "baby bump", from her social media networks. She also admitted to feeling pleased when a friend had lost her baby through miscarriage "because she isn't getting what I can't have". Acknowledging that these were "dreadful" thoughts, she also revealed the depth of jealousy and hatred she had experienced earlier on hearing the news of this pregnancy. With the loss of her friend's pregnancy, symmetry was restored. Sigrid then attempted to contextualise these norm-breaking emotions, which she saw as justifiable ("normal"), because of the very particular stresses associated with infertility: their resentfulness was understandable, granted the daily roller-coaster they had to endure and of which "most people" were oblivious. They were "not horrible people", she asserted; and, finally, she emphasised the beneficial aspects of having such OSGs as Stronger Together to assist in coping with "those rough days". No matter how "horrible" and transgressive they might feel, there were always others who understood them in this online space, ready to offer words of compassion, thus strengthening their shared identities and group consciousness. Sigrid's post reinforced the uniqueness of their lived experiences and the claim that only others with similar experiences could genuinely recognise their pain.

Concerning the theme of the pregnant other, Sophie gave an account in her online journal of an insensitive co-worker because she was "still in disbelief" and wanted to "vent this out". Explaining that there was no one else to whom she could tell this story who "would understand", this particular linguistic "move" and others like it (presumably) helped to produce a sense of solidarity amongst the participants on the site:

A co-worker was just sitting in the office discussing some business related stuff. Then he noticed I had a picture of my boys hanging on the wall so he started talking about them. He asked if we were going to have another baby … I responded that I was in no way in that mindset yet. He mentioned that he and his wife were completely happy with having two sons and they weren't planning any more kids, but she accidentally got pregnant with their daughter. OK no big deal, but then he says this:
'Me and my wife are the anti you. We had problems NOT staying pregnant! Haha, we actually called her Fertile Myrtle because she wouldn't quit getting pregnant!'
What the F am I supposed to say to that? I ended up saying, 'Um, yeah, I pretty much hate people like you' … he replied, 'Yeah, I know.' He obviously never knew how saying something like that could hurt me so bad and I know he didn't mean anything by it but shit man, think about what you are saying!!!!

Sophie was particularly dismayed over his lack of sensitivity, since he knew of her struggles with IF and IVF. She felt hurt by his raising the question of additional children, but also acknowledged that he probably "didn't mean anything by it". Such encounters might be regarded as banal and commonplace by others, but assumed special significance in the context of infertility. As exemplified in this situation, the women were often astonished and disappointed at the seeming failure of others to anticipate their feelings, to take their "role".

Undeserving Pregnant Others and Moral Outrage

Through their IF journeys, the women's attention was drawn anew to very particular observations of other mothers, including those they saw as underserving of motherhood. Many of these observations carried assumptions concerning the very poor parenting skills of mothers from low socio-economic backgrounds, and the limited life chances of their children, as we see in the following excerpt from Sophie's journal:

> Just yesterday while at Wal-Mart, I was stuck in an aisle with a 16 year old mom with three kids and I caught myself thinking, *Those poor children don't have a chance ... I should take them home and give them some love.* (Italics included)

Judgments were made about young single mothers and parents in unstable domestic situations that could have a damaging effect on their children—especially those characterised by joblessness, absent fathers and abusive partners. They railed against the injustice that these women could fall pregnant so easily, raise their children in socially and emotionally deprived environments and apparently not appreciate them. A week or so after her visit to the local Wal-Mart store, Sophie referred again to the image of the undeserving Wal-Mart mother. In a journal entry titled "Confused and sorta hurt", she related her sister's poor treatment of her daughter:

She had a hard time conceiving her daughter so we have always had a bond over that … She was so incredibly happy when Emma was a baby … and it seemed like she truly appreciated Emma. This last weekend it was like a completely different sister. She was so angry with Emma all the time, wouldn't stop yelling at her, constantly berated her about something she was doing (she's 3, so yeah, she does a lot of stupid things! She's a toddler for crying out loud!) I was in shock. I never thought I would see someone so close to me who had experienced pain with conceiving and someone who knows what I went through to treat a child like that! … She was acting like one of those women in Wal-Mart that is screaming at their kid and it makes you want to walk over and punch the mom and take the kid. MY SISTER WAS ONE OF THOSE PEOPLE!!!

Sophie explained her attempts to be "supportive" in case her sister had been going through a "hard time" in the lead up to the angry outbursts. However, she also told her that "'Children are a blessing and if you can't see that Emma is a precious gift, you should feel ashamed!'" Later, in the entry, she declared "if I went home and told my husband any of this he would look at me like I'm a crazy alien *so I just needed to vent it out here*" (Italics added). Here she asserted that the emotional terrain of infertility could not be traversed by those without lived experience of the condition because, in many situations, their concerns would appear "alien" to others (Barak et al. 2008). This move, like many similar "moves" made by the participants of Stronger Together, reinforced the uniqueness of the women's identities and their group consciousness, and also illustrated the process of triangulation.

A post made by Kerryn to the general discussion board conveyed the incredulity of many of the participants towards women they saw as undeserving mothers, especially when they fell pregnant very easily. In the midst of "dealing" with her IF treatment, Kerryn had received a text from DH's sister announcing her pregnancy. Exasperated, she posted: "Well that's just great"; the woman and her partner were "both jobless", lived with his father, and "to top it all off" she often phoned Kerryn when the partner was abusive. Why, she asked, are such people "blessed with a child?" As discussed in the previous chapter, many of these posts touched on such existential questions as why they themselves had been dealt the card of infertility when others not equipped for motherhood were "blessed" with children.

Returning to Patricia's journal, we see the theme of the "undeserving" pregnant other very distinctly. While pregnant during her fourth IVF cycle (a pregnancy she loses after several weeks), and feeling "scared shitless" about losing it, Patricia discovered that one of her closest friends, the mother of a two-year old, was pregnant again:

> And here's the kicker ... she's my age [early 40s] and was trying for one whole month! Here's the catch ... she was separated from her husband with a pending divorce for the past year! He walked out when the baby was 4 months. He refused to give her any money for the baby. They were in and out of court forever! She was a mess!
>
> ... Needless to say, she slept with her husband a few times since he came back home in May and wham, bam, thank you ma'am she is knocked up!

Given these circumstances, Patricia admitted not knowing "how to be happy for her":

> "I was there throughout the whole mess ... Why does God give babies to women that are staying in a horrible relationship with a piece of trash, yet keeps them out of the arms of women who are ready and willing to do anything to have them and have people in their lives to support this dream?"

This imponderable dilemma often intensified the pain of infertility:

> [I can't believe there's a God who could] be so cruel as to take this dream from me once again and yet give babies to the so many that are not prepared or equipped to have them ... There's the one with the deadbeat husband who got knocked up with the second kid and will be due about three weeks after me. I know our friendship will be over if I lose this baby. She will be the constant reminder of what I should have had. That's how cruel IF is. Not only is it breaking my heart ... it's making me feel like a failure to my DH, destroying friendships, making me regret my profession [teacher], making me feel like half a woman.

Feeling "like half a woman" encapsulates very poignantly the shame Patricia felt for failing to achieve motherhood, for failing to reach her potential. As Chase and Walker (2012, p. 740) argue, shame is revealed as "a sense of powerlessness and feeling small".

Not long afterwards, she received a message from her pregnant friend, saying she had miscarried: "I felt horrible and now started to worry that my anger … is going to cause karma to bite me in the ass this week at my RE apt." Patricia felt caught in an emotional crossfire. Drawing on the pioneering work of Arlie Hochschild (1979), she was trapped between "the normative and the experiential": between the "feeling rules" indicating the emotions we are expected to feel and express in particular social settings (i.e. in response to the news of a friend's pregnancy), and her actual experience of emotions (Illouz et al. 2014, p. 223). Fundamentally, then, her experience characterises the destabilisation of key relationships and emotional entrapment in the context of the infertility journey. The gap between "the normative and the experiential" is mediated through the process of emotion management, wherein individuals *work on* their feelings, as shown in numerous examples thus far. They might attempt to evoke or suppress particular feelings, or change the quality or degree of them, or challenge the feeling rules themselves, as we saw in Sigrid's post. However, managing the gap between the normative and experiential was exceedingly difficult for many Stronger Together participants, ensconced as most were in the "roller-coaster" ride of cheating hopes and repeated failures. We might surmise, then, that many of the women had to live with this "gap" while holding onto the dream of motherhood.

Conclusion

This chapter has examined the destabilisation of key relationships in the women's lives in the context of their experiences of infertility. We focused specifically on the stresses they encountered in their relationships with family, friends and work colleagues. We also considered posts that revealed the painful and conflicted feelings triggered by Mothers' Day celebrations, and the moral outrage directed to such "undeserving" pregnant others as teenage mothers, unemployed parents and those living in chaotic domestic situations.

The hurts occasioned by fertile others' apparent lack of consideration for the pain and distress caused by infertility, and the news of others' pregnancies were amongst the most frequently discussed stresses in the online space. As demonstrated in the journal entries and posts we analysed, the women were often disturbed and guilt-ridden by their reactions to others' pregnancies, and overwhelmed by the depth of sadness generated by such news. Acutely aware of the gap between the normative expectations of joy and congratulations, at these times, and the "experiential" realm of ambivalence, sadness and shame over their childlessness, many of the women ruminated over their emotional reactions in the online space. One woman described herself as feeling like a "crappy friend", and another that she felt like "half a woman". The women were often troubled by the question of whether their unwelcome feelings were legitimate. We argued that these ruminations seemed to produce a form of emotional entrapment that demanded emotional regulation and emotional justice.

In this chapter, we also continued our observations of the "triangulation" of the women's key relationships and intimacies. This process indicates a re-grouping of the women's key intimacies across three intersecting points: relationships with family, friends and work colleagues; their partners; and their online relationships. The women often commented that their online interactions offered a level of "recognition" (Frost 2016) more meaningful than the support offered by offline others who lacked firsthand experience of infertility. As a consequence, the women's relationships with their significant (offline) others were often sidelined in the presence of their online connections. Linda's post, which welcomes a newcomer to the site, captured the sentiments that the women frequently expressed about their involvement in the OSG:

> You definitely came to the right place … I hope you are able to find the support you need from people who are walking in your shoes. This has been one of my greatest supports to get me through some dark times.

References

Barak, A., Boniel-Nissim, M., & Suler, J. (2008). Fostering Empowerment in Online Support Groups. *Computers in Human Behavior, 24*(5), 1867–1883.

Chase, E., & Walker, R. (2012). The Co-Construction of Shame in the Context of Poverty: Beyond a Threat to the Social Bond. *Sociology, 47*(4), 739–754.

Clarke, C. (1997). *Misery and Company: Sympathy in Everyday Life*. Chicago: University of Chicago Press.

Dermott, E., & Seymour, J. (2011). Developing "Displaying Families": A Possibility for the Future of the Sociology of Personal Life. In E. Dermott & J. Seymour (Eds.), *Displaying Families: A New Concept for the Sociology of Family Life* (pp. 3–18). Basingstoke; New York: Palgrave Macmillan.

Frost, L. (2016). Exploring the Concepts of Recognition and Shame for Social Work. *Journal of Social Work, 30*(4), 431–446.

Harkness, S. K., & Hitlin, S. (2014). Morality and the Emotions. In J. E. Stets & J. H. Turner (Eds.), *Handbook of the Sociology of Emotions* (Vol. II, pp. 451–471). Dordrecht, Netherlands: Springer.

Hochschild, A. R. (1979). Emotion Work, Feeling Rules, and Social Structure. *American Journal of Sociology, 85*(3), 551–575.

Hunt, S. J. (2017). *The Life Course: A Sociological Introduction*. London; New York: Palgrave Macmillan.

Illouz, E. (2003). *Oprah Winfrey and the Glamour of Misery*. New York: Columbia University Press.

Illouz, E. (2007). *Cold Intimacies: The Making of Emotional Capitalism*. Cambridge, UK: Polity Press.

Illouz, E. (2008). *Saving the Modern Soul: Therapy, Emotions, and the Culture of Self-Help*. Berkeley, CA: University of California Press.

Illouz, E., Gilon, D., & Shachak, M. (2014). Emotions and Cultural Theory. In J. E. Stets & J. H. Turner (Eds.), *Handbook of the Sociology of Emotions* (Vol. II, pp. 221–244). Dordrecht, Netherlands: Springer.

Karp, D. (2001). *The Burden of Sympathy: How Families Cope with Mental Illness*. Oxford; New York: Oxford University Press.

Lively, K. J., & Weed, E. A. (2014). Emotion Management: Sociological Insight into What, How, Why, and to What End? *Emotion Review, 6*(3), 202–207.

Pennebaker, J. W., & Evans, J. F. (2014). *Expressive Writing: Words that Heal*. Enumclaw, WA: Idyll Arbor.

Pennebaker, J. W., & Smyth, J. (2016). *Opening Up by Writing It Down: The Healing Power of Expressive Writing*. New York: Guilford.

Silva, J. (2013). *Coming Up Short: Working-Class Adulthood in an Age of Uncertainty*. New York: Oxford University Press.

6

Partnering the Infertile: The Impact of Infertility on Women's Spousal Relationships

Paulina Billett

"Infertility is horrible … and it may end up ruining my marriage (which is only 4 months old). I may do this round of IVF (if the DH will still do it) and then call it quits. I don't want to live like this."—Patricia.

Introduction

The journal entry from which the above excerpt originated is highly significant. In it, Patricia describes in detail the almost love-hate relationship which many women hold with their infertility. Patricia opens her journal by describing this as the "worst day", she recounts advice from doctors which leads to attempting treatment she is not comfortable with, but feels obliged to try, as her partner may decide to strop treatment if she is unwilling "to try every-

P. Billett (✉)
La Trobe University, Melbourne, Australia
e-mail: p.billett@latorbe.edu.au

© The Author(s) 2019
P. Billett, A.-M. Sawyer, *Infertility and Intimacy in an Online Community*,
Palgrave Macmillan Studies in Family and Intimate Life,
https://doi.org/10.1057/978-1-137-44981-8_6

thing that the RE [reproductive endocrinologist] suggested". Patricia's entry relates a truly isolating experience, one where women "have to do everything" while husbands seem to do very little. This type of entry was not uncommon, and through our research we saw a number of examples which described the sometimes uncomfortable navigation many women undertake between their own and their partner's wishes and expectations. For many, these expectations were vastly different (or were perceived to be by the women) and were often the source of friction in the couple's relationship. However, when the couple's expectations aligned, the relationship provided what can be argued to be the single most important source of support during testing, diagnosis and treatment and helped women to cope better with the demands of protocols and the disappointments of failed attempts.

Understanding the role which relationships play in the lives of infertile women is essential. As we have previously demonstrated, the support we receive from our relationships (be it our relationship to ourselves or to others) has the power to affect our capacity to deal effectively, even creatively, with life's many challenges. In Chap. 3, we dealt with the first of the three relationship nodes (online friendships) and Chap. 5 discussed the second node (relationships with offline others). In this chapter, we deal with the third node of our relationship triangle: the couple relationship. In particular, we seek to explore how intimate partner relationships affect and enable the ability of infertile women to deal with the realities which treatment and the possible loss of motherhood entails.

While infertility is often viewed as a woman's problem, past research has shown that infertility is not an individual experience, but instead it is a shared experience between a couple (Greil 1997; Savitz-Smith 2003; Schmidt et al. 2005). As such, while this book is primarily an exploration of women's experiences of infertility, we felt it relevant to discuss intimate partner relationships in terms of its meaning in the women's journeys.

Relational Uncertainty, Partner Interference and Boundary Turbulence

Our research, like others before it (e.g. see Steuber and Solomon 2008 and 2012), found that the roller-coaster of emotion experienced during the infertility journey creates a shift in the couple's relationship leading to what Solomon and Knobloch (2004) term relational turbulence. Relational turbulence refers to how "relationship transitions [particularly life altering ones such as infertility] polarize emotions and cognitive appraisals and disrupt the exchange of messages between partners" (Solomon 2016, p. 1). Relational turbulence results in higher levels of stress for the couple emphasised by relational uncertainty in the form of uncertainty on the partner's commitment to the treatment and resolution of their infertile status.

The experience of infertility is a tough challenge for most infertile couples, who unlike "normal" couples, report the need to confront "new realities"; cope with financial pressures from treatment; learn a new "language" based on medical terminology and discourse; consider existential questions including the stresses of failed attempts, choices about changing or ending treatment, as well as contending with ethical questions such as what to do with unused embryos after treatment (see Matthews and Matthews 1986; Savitz-Smith 2003; Schmidt et al. 2005). This time of relational turbulence, requires couples to "re-adjust" to these new realities leading to periods of intense uncertainty, resulting in some women experiencing doubts about their partner's investment in treatment and its goals.

Unsurprisingly, the intense feelings of anger, resentment, depression and confusion experienced through the journey of infertility and fertility treatment can severely undermine a couple's relationship. In particular, reactions to the difficulties of this journey provoke intense reactions (both positive and negative) and create a veritable roller-coaster, one which couples reported feeling unable to "get off" no matter how hard they tried. For most, this was a difficult situation, with women frequently questioning their partners' commitment to treatment (and at times the relationship itself) and reporting intense feelings of isolation from their partner.

In terms of support, expectations and feelings of isolation, the earlier years seemed to present the most intense challenge for couples and led to greater levels of relational uncertainty. In the beginning, couples faced with the painful inability to conceive are confronted with an uncertain future which they must now negotiate. Once investigations begin, they are put through countless invasive procedures, which may or may not shed light on their condition. Upon diagnosis couples must make the choice of continuing to try "alone" or submitting to further tests and incredibly expensive procedures, such as IVF, which have unclear success rates. For women, this situation is even more challenging, as the majority of exploratory investigations, testing and subsequent procedures are undertaken on the female.

A consequence of this intense focus on the female body is that infertility is constructed as a woman's problem, which marginalises men from fertility treatment (Malik and Coulson 2008b; Hanna and Gough 2016, 2017). Previous literature on infertile couples has discussed that the feminine focus of infertility has rendered fertility treatment as a "second job" for women, (see for example Steuber and Solomon 2008) who take on the majority of the "infertility burden" including coordination of fertility related activities; such as timing of intercourse, channelling of large portions of the couple's funds into testing and procedures and the reshaping of everyday life to suit treatment cycles, while men see their primary role as one of support (Hanna and Gough 2016, 2017). This inevitably results in increased levels of anxiety due to misunderstandings and incongruent expectations, intensified levels of partner interference, which exacerbate existing difficulties, and higher levels of relational uncertainty. This heightened level of anxiety is further impacted by private boundary turbulence as the couple navigates the reshaping of boundaries and the sharing of intimate, and often sensitive, information between the partners and with others.

It is not surprising that, excluding discussion of treatment, the stresses of infertility and its impact on the couple's relationship was one of the most often encountered discussions in the women's journals. Journaling about the couple's relationship seems to take three forms; journaling about supportive behaviour, journaling to vent about what was perceived to be unsupportive behaviour or discussing protective attitudes and behaviours towards their partner. We deal with each in turn.

Feeling Supported

Infertile couples frequently do not receive support from friends or family because they often feel uncomfortable discussing their personal journey with others. As we saw in our discussion in Chap. 5, fear of being

misunderstood or judged will keep many couples silent about their struggle. As a result, partners in a relationship commonly become each other's
most important form of support (Abbey et al. 1995). For women undergoing fertility treatment, a partner's "appropriate" reaction to events and
acceptance of partner interference during their journey can present a
form of validation of their own feelings. Congruence in a couple's
appraisal of the challenges posed by infertility lead to higher levels of
marital adjustment and can help to reduce the stress they experience and
increase the couple's ability to manage this highly taxing situation
(Peterson et al. 2003). Not surprisingly, the joy felt by women when their
partner assumed a congruent stance, and/or accepted partner interference in relation to treatment, was palpable. Many of the women rejoiced
in what they considered to be the most supportive aspects of their partner's behaviours, such as taking time to research treatments and conditions, taking vitamins and other medication; demonstrating supportive
behaviours such as attending appointments, and showing willingness to
discuss fertility issues; and tangible displays of emotions, such as showing
happiness at successes or displaying frustration due to failure. For the
women of Stronger Together, these simple cues meant that their partner
was as vested in their journey as they were, giving them a source of comfort and reassurance against an often unstable situation.

Sadly, while the entries which described supportive attitudes by partners were few, those that contained accounts of partner supportive behaviour were always greatly valued and celebrated. Of the entries made by
the women, Joan's journal stands out. Joan and her husband Richard had
been trying to conceive for around five years before joining Stronger
Together. Throughout her two years of writing, Joan's husband Richard
was often praised in her journal for his loving and considerate attitude to
their struggle. To Joan, Richard often showed responsiveness towards
their ups and downs, tolerated her demands, and is complimented by his
wife for showing emotions such as happiness, excitement and sadness.
His positive reactions and indeed acceptance of partner interference in
their daily routine were seen by Joan as proof that he cares and that he is
vested in the process just as much as she is. For example, in one of her
entries, Joan shares her excitement at finally having a positive result in her

ovulation test. As she suffers from PCOS and does not ovulate often on her own, she was excited at being able to share the good news with her husband. Joan shares that after texting him the news, he replied "saying that it definitely put a bounce in his step!"

Her journal moves on to comment on the ensuing "on demand" sexual activity (which is perceived by most women as further evidence of support) and medical symptoms which may spell out a pregnancy. At a later date, his positive reaction, once again, to ovulation is commented on by Joan, who writes:

> I got a positive LH test on Wednesday afternoon. DH was home, so he and I rejoiced a bit.

In each of Joan's entries, appearance of a "team effort" is demonstrated by each partner having internalised and enacted their expected "role"— Joan shoulders the responsibility of testing and setting the timing, while Richard performs emotionally and sexually when prompted by Joan.

For others, such as Lilly, the fact that her partner is able to feel the pain of childlessness like she does is important. In one of her entries she mentions her husband's sadness at hearing of new pregnancies and his angst at how this may upset her:

> DH and I sat down after I found out about his cousin's pregnancy. I was so angry with him for not telling me earlier! I just wanted to rage!!!!! He told me that he didn't want to tell me because it had really upset him, and he was so worried about how I would feel about it all after our loss. All my anger vanished, I just wanted to hug him so tight ...

Joan and Lilly are not alone in perceiving certain action and reactions as evidence of support. On a thread post, Kerry comments with excitement on her husband's appropriate response, and writes that she "could not have picked out a better partner for this journey ..." She goes on to suggest that his supportive behaviour, including his willingness to attend doctor's appointments, work extra hours to meet financial demands and "let me hang out in my pjs all day when I just don't feel like facing the day after my BFNs ..." are evidence of his support for the journey they have undertaken. Kerry's husband, like Joan's and Lilly's, is appropriately enacting the role of supporter, one who is willing to limit his own role to that of follower and protector while accepting his partner's guidance in the process. In short, for these women, as for many others who responded on these threads, their husbands' supportive behaviours are evidence that they are vested in the process, making their struggled shared rather than one-sided.

However, the need to maintain a high level of support among the partners can be a high impact stressor and has been suggested as a predictor of poor marital outcomes (see for example Schmidt et al. 2005). It has been documented by those such as Hanna and Gough (2016, 2017) that like women, men also find the experience of infertility as deeply isolating. Often men find it hard to discuss emotions about infertility, even with other men in similar situations. Men, in their studies often felt at a loss as to how to help their female partners and often deployed stereotyped explanations of the differences between masculinity and femininity, including the need to prioritise their partner's needs above their own, as reasoning for their perceived shortcoming.

However, the pressure of always being "there" often became too much for even the most supportive of men. According to the women of Stronger Together, the ensuing response was for men to simply "switch off" and attempt to withdraw from the onslaught of the infertility roller-coaster. For the majority of women, this shift in attention was often seen as abandonment, leading to anger and resentment. Inevitably, posts and journals were often dedicated to venting about a partner's behaviour rather than singing their praises.

When Support Fails

Given the gender role expectations and the level of invasiveness of treatments, it is reasonable to suspect that males and females may have different responses to fertility treatment. For many women, the inability to fulfil societal roles and social comparison to women who have children can be a major contributor to depression (Newton et al. 1999); men, on the other hand, seem to see infertility as an unfortunate but resolvable issue (Greil 1991). The divide between a couple's perceptions of the impact of infertility, as well as difference in the reactions between males and females, can create a gulf of understanding between the partners (Chachamovich et al. 2010). These differences were frequently perceived by women as unsupportive behaviour.

As discussed previously, women often perceived supportive attitudes as those in which their partner's reactions mirrored their own. When a couple's attitudes did not mirror one another, this was perceived as evidence of lack of support and was often a precursor to arguments and the inevitable, though usually temporary, breakdown of communication between the couple.

For many women, the lack of communication with their partner was a major source of angst. This was particularly troublesome during times of treatment, where much of the women's attention was engaged in medical procedures and the process of conception. Lack of communication during this time in particular made the experience far more stressful for the women undergoing it. Mary discusses in her journal how her husband's approach to infertility is making her feel isolated and reinforces her need for support at this time:

> I need to know that he is with me 100% in mind and body, it's not a lot to ask for …

This resentment is mirrored by Catherine in response to another member's discussion, by highlighting her husband's lack of sensitivity to her struggle with the statement: "My DH just doesn't get it either." She goes on to quote what she felt was a particularly insensitive remark (regarding his perception of her obsession) as evidence of his lack of support.

The lack of support from a partner can be even more stressful for women who feel misunderstood by their partner in their search for an answer to their condition. The amount of time spent by many women researching their condition, its treatment and possible outcomes was frequently perceived by partners as an obsession. This unsurprisingly was often a point of friction for the couple. While for many of the women attempting to find answers became a compulsion, for their partners their perpetual engagement in the world of infertility was an obsession which needed to be controlled. Time and time again, we encountered journals which lamented a partner's annoyance at the women's monotonous musings on treatment. These rebuffs often caused much sadness, as the apparent rejection was perceived as a lack of interest in having a baby and a withdrawal of emotional support. This was very evident in Mary's journal, where she discusses her husband's disengagement in their treatment through many of her entries. One in particular shows the depth of emotion that her partner's disinterest conveys to her:

> I said to him, are you excited about next week, YESSSSSSS in a long droned tone he said. I said to him why are you being like that—like you don't care, you need to give me 100% support and I need to feel your excitement, I also told him that I felt he was being negative and that we should be going into this with full excitement and 100% support for each other, he then got really defensive and told me, I was obsessed, and he didn't need to hear about it every day …

Mary also reports her husband's labelling of her need to discuss infertility as an obsession as a hurtful accusation, in response to a thread discussing partners' reactions to women's journeys. She writes that her partner often became frustrated by her constant discussion of IVF and infertility, telling her that she tended to over-analyse and needed to take just one day at a time. She concludes with the statement "THAT WAS HARD …"

Other women, such as Bethany, reacted with anger, rather than sadness at their husband's inability to show empathy. In a furious entry in which she discusses her partner's lack of support, both emotionally and financially, she closes with:

> You have to jack off in a cup. I have to be molested and probed. Wanna trade places?

To Bethany, her husband's failure to appreciate what she is going through is a source of anger and disappointment. She, as many other women, feels that the unfair burden placed on her body should be taken in consideration by her partner and was incensed when she felt attacked and misunderstood.

Deciding if and when to pause or end treatment can also be a major stressor for the couple, presenting a period of intense relational uncertainty. Undergoing fertility treatment is an ongoing stressful situation. For most women, the desire to continue treatment is based on their fear of giving up too early. The question of giving up was one often discussed in discussion boards and journals, particularly after failed treatment cycles. In these journals and posts the women often considered the possibility that pregnancy may never ensue. The message most frequently heard was: I don't want to give up because success could be just around the corner. In her post, Abigail discusses her desire to stop treatment but is concerned that "what if the next time is THE ONE!". Jacinta echoes this in her own post where she laments her devastation at yet another BFN and states "I don't want to give up, but it is hard" and "I am too scared to stop."

The decision to stop treatment is invariably a difficult one, even when this is for a short while. What complicates this even further is that infertility, unlike other illnesses, does not allow for unilateral decision-making and partners often found themselves at different levels of acceptance and understanding of their childlessness (see Leigh 2016). Penelope's post encapsulates this battle where she states that at 36 her husband is ready to give up, but she remains unsure as she knows that at 36 time is not on her side, and poses the question: "How do I know when enough is enough?"

While it is usually the female in the partnership who may not want to move on from treatment, at times it may be the male partner who may want to continue treatment or indeed "regress" to an earlier stage. Such was the experience of Jessie. After having tried for over a year to have a child, Jessie and her partner decided to move on to adopt, rather than to put their energy into continued diagnosis and treatment. During their adoption journey, they became pregnant, but unfortunately experienced the devastation of a miscarriage. They decided to attempt conceiving again. However, after four unsuccessful months, Jessie decided that she had had enough and wanted to once again begin the process of adoption.

She was left stunned when her husband professed a desire not to move on, but instead to begin testing in order to "search for answers":

> So DH now doesn't want to adopt ... WTF I thought we were moving forward with this! I want to have a child, and I don't want to do this SHIT again!!!! I'm over the doctors, needles and the endless watching of the pee stick but no, now he wants to go back and begin looking for answers again! Like we haven't tried!!!!

It is unsurprising that so many of those undergoing fertility treatment find it so difficult to end their journey. Stories of success from group members coupled with the exaltation of advances by "claim makers" can make a couple uncertain whether to continue or discontinue their IF journeys. For many of the women, it is the "what if" which keeps them going: the expectation that one day they will achieve a family which keeps them pushing beyond physical, mental and emotional endurance. While many felt drained emotionally and physically by the never-ending cycle of testing, treatment and failure to conceive, their desperation to achieve "normalcy" through creating a family added a further level of pressure to already overstretched nerves.

As a result, infertility is more than a medical condition. Infertility affects how individuals feel about themselves, their relationships and their perspectives on life (Hart 2002). For the women of Stronger Together ceasing treatment was more than just a simple choice. It was the admittance of surrender, accepting that "normalcy" was beyond reach and seen as failure to persevere in the face of adversity.

As the years wore on and as the women developed a better understanding of procedures, and indeed grew more accustomed to failure, their need for reassurance also diminished making their partner's response less problematic. This finding is not uncommon; Gerrity (2001) suggests that the marital stress experienced by couples undergoing treatment may differ through different stages of the infertility journey and may ease as times progresses. One thing, however, remained relatively constant and changed little in terms of the women's reaction: their need to protect their partner from the trials of the infertility journey at all costs.

To Love and Protect

As discussed previously, women and men seem to take two different roles during the infertility journey—that of leader or supporter. While women almost exclusively appear to take the lead (meaning that they shoulder most of responsibility for testing and treatment during the infertility journey), at times they also take the role of supporter. This was particularly true of women attempting to shield their partners from the trials of the infertility journey. Protection of one's partners took two basic forms: protection from performance anxiety and loss of spontaneity; and, protection from the stress associated with the ongoing fertility treatment, including the discovery of male factor. We review each in turn.

Loss of Spontaneity and Pleasure in the Couple Relationship

An important theme that was raised by the women was the loss of spontaneity and pleasure in the couple relationship. As entries progressed, and the women delved deeper into the world of fertility treatment, it was clear that life was very quickly reduced to monotony, something which many of the women deeply regretted. All those who shared their stories with us felt that their couple relationship had been greatly affected by the demands of treatment and a number of them voiced their need to take a break during the years in which they continued to journal and post on the general thread. For the majority of women, the feeling of being out of control was felt not only in terms of their own bodies, but also in terms of their couple relationship. A number of journals and posts discussed the impact that infertility and the treatment journey were having on their relationship. As time progressed a number of the women began to ask themselves if it was time to "take a break". This was often suggested as a way of regaining control, as well as allowing the couple some room to reconnect at a level other than conception.

An example can be seen in the following excerpt from Mary's journal who, after a number of unsuccessful attempts, discusses the impact the journey is having on herself and her husband and the need to take a break:

As a matter of fact, my DH and I have discussed stopping this stuff altogether for a couple of months if we are not successful this month. It is just getting so exhausting and we both need a break and time to enjoy life! I will be sad, and may not be able to stop trying for more than a month, but I just can't deal with all of the bad news anymore.

However, it was not until the end of that particular cycle, and the crushing negative pregnancy test, that Mary felt ready to take time away from treatment, as she writes:

Well I have NOTHING good to report. Christmas will be a sad one as I had feared. I plan on buying a few bottles of wine to drink over Christmas and New Years and just try to say goodbye to 2011 ... a year filled with horrible shots, pills, suppositories, early morning doctor appointments, tons of weight gain and not feeling attractive, mood swings, arguing with DH, tears, fears, headaches, acupuncture, cancelled plans because of how I was feeling, anger and some of the saddest news anyone can get (BFNs) ... We plan on taking a break for a month or two at least before we decide if we can do this again. I hope that I have it in me, but I worry about becoming a totally depressed wife that my DH will not want to be around!

She once again writes after having taken time off and recounts the benefits and her subsequent trepidation at returning to fertility treatment, reflecting:

Well this month has been quite enjoyable so far.
Enjoyed some wine, good food, laughs with my DH!
Enjoyed not feeling exhausted, moody, emotional!
Enjoyed having the energy to get back to the gym for the first time in over a year (although I still despise the gym ....it is a necessary evil!)
Enjoyed having sex because I wanted to and not having to worry about abstaining before a procedure or being too tired to do anything.
Enjoyed LIFE!
AND THEN IT HAPPENED!
THE TWO BIG BOXES OF MEDS SHOWED UP AT THE DOOR!
REMINDING ME THAT THIS NIGHTMARE IS HARDLY OVER!

Similar to Mary, Erin also recounted in her journal her positive experiences after making the difficult decision to take time off:

I have been feeling so much better since we made the decision to take a break. I'm still working on this round of Clomid, but I'm not thinking about it much at all. Occasionally, my brain will try to tell me that it is working, but I remind myself about the ultrasounds I have had recently and tell myself that there is almost no way it would work. My DH is having some issues with his medication as well, so it is nice to be on a break for a while until we get that straightened out. Our focus has just been on each other … not any of the crap that has been stressing us out. It's so nice! I'm reminded of when we were first married and didn't really worry about anything. We just took it all one day at a time.

Having time away also provided an opportunity to work on other aspects of their relationships. This was particularly true of their sex lives, which were often negatively affected by the experience of infertility and fertility treatment. Upon reading the women's journal entries and posts, it became clear that due to the demands of treatment, sexual intimacy took an obligatory character which was focused on conception alone, rather than something to be shared and enjoyed by the couple.

Sexual activity during treatments is always a difficult affair. Whether it is in the initial testing phase or during treatment with Clomid, IUI, IVF or other methods, medical protocols require sex to be timed to cycles during times of ovulation, pills or shots set by doctors and other treating clinicians. For the couple "baby dancing", as they call sexual activity, often becomes a chore, something which must be gotten over with rather than something which is intimate and pleasurable. This situation was often described as highly distressing to the couple. Joan explains that she and her husband often found it difficult to have intercourse on a regular basis, partly due to low libido on her part and partly due to the stresses of infertility. She goes on to recount that she is trying to get "interested in it" (though she does not explain what this may entail) so they can begin having intercourse every day. She concludes her entry by stating:

> I know it'll only be a week or so of BDing every day, but man does that seem daunting!

Performance anxiety also became an issue for some men, rendering them unable to perform and causing further stress and strain on the couple. In her post Megan relates to others her concern over her partner's inability to perform and particularly "not being able to perform and finish" when they only have "today and tomorrow". She states that she has asked her partner to "see a doctor".

Megan's partner is not alone in his response to the overwhelming pressure for sex on demand. In the replies to this and similar posts, a number of women discussed performance anxiety as an issue for their partners. Once again, taking on their role as leaders in their IF journey, women asked for advice as to how to rekindle passion in the bedroom, with answers ranging from ensuring date nights, taking time off for holidays to a number of women advising others to take on the responsibilities for treatment (such as monitoring ovulation) and keeping their partner as "shielded" as possible from these concerns. This, it was discussed, would take the pressure off their partner, allowing the man to regain enjoyment in sex. Such was Jane's suggestion to one woman's post, where she recommends not telling her partner but, instead, taking on the role of instigator. In her reply to the post, she details how she let her partner think that "he was this super-hot stud that I couldn't keep my hands off ALL of the time", even though "It was a little tiresome for me."

Another suggestion given by Wanda to the same post mirrored Jane's reply. In it, Wanda suggests "not [to] make a big deal about it ... I said that it was just part of the process and the same way I had to take drugs to ovulate, he could take drugs for it too". In the end she relates how she not only solicited the prescription for erection pills from her doctor, but also filled the prescription "to save any embarrassment for my husband".

One of the curious themes in these discussions, as well as in many other similar discussions, is that while the women acknowledge their own discomfort and openly discussed their anxieties, their desire to conceive drove them to disavow their own needs in the hope of protecting their partner. These discussions also exemplify that, for women, conception is still very much a "woman's" domain. Whether or not they are the source of infertility, they felt obliged to lessen the burden on their partners by taking over responsibilities for treatment and absorbing the burden of reproduction in the hope that this cycle may prove to be their last.

Protecting from Disappointment and Judgement

For many couples, it is the male rather than the female who is faced with infertility. In fact, Resolve, the US based national infertility association suggests that around 30% of all the cases of infertility involve partly or exclusively male factor due to "problems such as structural abnormalities, sperm production disorders, ejaculatory disturbances and immunologic disorders" (Resolve website). Nonetheless, society and medical practice continues to construct infertility as a woman's issue (Carmeli and Birenbaum-Carmeli 1994). It is not surprising that a diagnosis of infertility may come as a shock to many males, who often have not considered this possibility. For many men, there is a feeling of shame at being labelled infertile, for after all, male fertility is tightly linked to ideas of virility in most societies. Hanna and Gough (2016, 2017) found that participants in their studies often suggested that aspects of their masculinity had been compromised by infertility and saw it as invading all aspects of their lives. For many men, being "outed" as infertile was a difficult experience, and one which limited women's ability to share with others in an open manner. Peter's reaction to his wife's disclosure of their test results to her brother further supports this. Elisabeth writes in her journal how she is particularly close to her brother and thus felt comfortable confiding in him about the poor results she and Peter had received on their last semen analysis. Peter was greatly angered by this and Elisabeth writes that it is because:

> He says that it's an uncomfortable thing for guys, that it's a judgement on their virility.

In this instance of intimate boundary turbulence, the couple must come to terms with the impact of infertility on the male partner. In short, they must acknowledge that infertility is more than just a woman's problem and renegotiate what can and what cannot be permissibly discussed with others. Interestingly, most women were highly concerned about their partner's reaction in finding out that they were unable to provide their wife with a child. Unlike their fears of becoming "unwanted" because of their inability to produce a child for their husbands, women's reactions to diagnosis of male factor brought an intense preoccupation centred on their partner's mental wellbeing and the best manner to "treat" their infertility. Patricia gives a despairing account of the difficulties she faced in attempting to support her husband's struggle:

> I feel horrible for him too because he was told he has a very low sperm count and he is trying to do anything he can (bought boxers, eating foods that are supposed to help improve sperm count, etc …) to make this happen. It has to feel disheartening to him as well. I am sure we are both feeling like failures.

In a similar journal entry, Elisabeth expresses concern for her husband's wellbeing and discusses her attempts to shield him from her disappointment. In one such entry, she writes:

> I know he already feels bad enough as it is … I don't want him to feel like I'm blaming him, so I just sort of get quiet and crumple inside …

Further to protecting their partners from the anxiety of the male factor diagnosis, many of the women took on the role of protector from what they perceived to be personal attacks from friends and family. At times, parents, siblings, friends and even colleagues were discussed as having crossed the line when discussing men's infertility.

Feelings of sadness, anger and resentment were further complicated when they involved their partners. Unwaveringly, all posts and journal entries made by the women which dealt with this topic used language which showed a high degree of protectiveness over their partner. An example of this is Joan's anger at her mother's discussion about her husband's depression. In a scathing journal entry on her mother's interfering ways, she recounts how her mother's "instant reaction to the comment of my hubby being sad/depressed about the IF … is to diagnose the problem" (something that her mother blames on her husband's urinary tract infection). She ends her journal by stating, "Like we hadn't thought of that ourselves?"

Trudy's post provides another example. When her boss suggests that she would get pregnant if she "had sex with a real man", her reply is indignant. She firstly clarifies that her husband "is not the issue" (thus verifying his virility) and then suggests that her husband is "a really manly man". One interesting aspect about this post is that Trudy seems to be unconcerned with the level of inappropriateness displayed by her boss. However, she is incensed at the insinuation that her husband is not a "real" man.

For a few men, their infertility meant that they would never be able to produce a biological child. In cases such as these, the only options are either adoption or to take the more contentious approach of making use of a sperm donation. While for a number of men this was a perfectly acceptable option; for others, having a genetic link (and, thus having the ultimate proof of virility) is too significant, thus they are categorically against these options. The intense resistance of some partners drove women to consider an all or nothing approach. One such example is Tina, who, when advising another member of the community how to convince her husband that sperm donation may in fact be a viable option, suggests that "you can make the choice that if one can't be the biological parent, then neither of you will and you could adopt, or use a donor embryo …". In short, many women would rather sacrifice their own "genetic legacy" in order to secure their partner's agreement for the use of donor embryo or adoption.

Interestingly, egg donation and embryo adoption were seen as far less contentious. For many women with low ovarian reserves or low-quality eggs, embryo adoption or egg donation was felt to be a viable way of achieving pregnancy. A number of posts discussed men's much more relaxed attitudes towards adoption of a child or embryo and egg donation. This seems to be due to the stigma attached to male infertility, and these solutions afforded men protection in the form of secrecy of parental genetic identification.

Conclusion

The journey of the couples of Stronger Together was an eye-opening and, at times, heart-wrenching experience. It was hard not to feel deeply moved by the stories we read and the struggles these women and their partners faced. What these stories, as well as countless others demonstrate, is that infertility is a major life disruptor, which has deep effects on those who are intimately involved in it. The stories provided by the women further support current literature which suggests that the experience of infertility is not one-sided, or a "woman's journey", but is in fact a struggle faced by the couple, who must somehow overcome the devastation of diagnosis and unify as a team, to confront an uncertain future fraught with much sorrow and disappointment, in the hope of one day conceiving their much longed-for child. For women, this struggle is doubly hard, as they often feel isolated and seek solace and comfort in their partners, who may not fully understand their needs. Simultaneously, women also feel the need to support and protect their partners from the everyday stresses of the infertility journey as well as protect them from what they perceive as a brutal and uncompromising world.

No matter where in their journey couples found themselves, relationships were always affected by the journey of infertility. However, not all was lost: while this journey was difficult and trying for all, many couples were able to see the benefits gained from their difficult journey. A number of stories demonstrate that, while the journey to conception was indeed paved with many trials, this only made their relationships with their partners stronger. This finding is not unique. Other research, such as that conducted in Denmark by Schmidt et al. (2005), also suggests that while the journey of infertility may be disruptive to a couple, their relationship is often made stronger by the experience.

References

Abbey, A., Andrews, F. M., & Halman, J. L. (1995). Provision and Receipt of Social Support and Disregard: What Is Their Impact on the Marital Life Quality of Infertile and Fertile Couples? *Journal of Personality and Social Psychology, 68*(3), 455–469.

Carmeli, S., & Birenbaum-Carmeli, D. (1994). The Predicament of Masculinity: Towards Understanding the Male's Experience of Infertility Treatments. *Sex Roles, 30*(9–10), 663–677.

Chachamovich, R. L., Chachamovich, J. E., Ezer, H., Fleck, M. P., Knauth, D. R., & Pandolfi Passos, E. (2010). Agreement on Perceptions of Quality of

Life in Couples Dealing with Infertility. *Journal of Obstetric, Gynecologic, & Neonatal Nursing, 39*(5), 557–565.

Gerrity, D. A. (2001). Five Medical Treatment Stages of Infertility: Implications for Counselors. *Family Journal, 9*(2), 140–150.

Greil, A. L. (1991). *Not Yet Pregnant: Infertile Couples in Contemporary America.* New Brunswick: Rutgers University Press.

Greil, A. L. (1997). Infertility and Psychological Distress: A Critical Review of the Literature. *Social Science & Medicine, 45*(11), 1679–1704.

Hanna, E., & Gough, B. (2016). Emoting Infertility Online: A Qualitative Analysis of Men's Forum Posts. *Health, 20*(4), 363–382.

Hanna, E., & Gough, B. (2017). Men's Accounts of Infertility Within Their Intimate Partner Relationships: An Analysis of Online Forum Discussions. *Journal of Reproductive and Infant Psychology, 35*(2), 150–158.

Hart, V. A. (2002). Infertility and the Role of Psychotherapy. *Issues in Metal Health Nursing, 23*(1), 31–41.

Leigh, J. (2016). *Avalanche: A Love Story.* Melbourne: Penguin Group Australia.

Malik, S. H., & Coulson, N. S. (2008a). Computer-Mediated Infertility Support Groups: An Exploratory Study of Online Experiences. *Patient Education and Counseling, 73*(1), 105–113.

Malik, S. H., & Coulson, N. S. (2008b). The Male Experience of Infertility: A Thematic Analysis of an Online Infertility Support Group Bulletin Board. *Journal of Reproductive and infant psychology, 26*(1), 18–30.

Matthews, R., & Matthews, A. M. (1986). Infertility and Involuntary Childlessness: Transition to Non-Parenthood. *Journal of Marriage and the Family, 48*(3), 641–649.

Newton, C. R., Sherrad, W., & Glavac, I. (1999). The Fertility Problem Inventory: Measuring Perceived Fertility Related Stress. *Fertility and Sterility, 72*(1), 54–62.

Peterson, B. D., Newton, C. R., Rosen, K. H., & Skaggs, G. E. (2003). Examining Congruence Between Partners' Perceived Infertility-Related Stress and Its Relationship to Marital Adjustment and Depression in Infertile Couples. *Family Process, 42*(1), 59–70.

Savitz-Smith, J. (2003). Couples Undergoing Fertility Treatment: Implications for Counselors. *The Family Journal, 11*(4), 383–386.

Schmidt, L., Bjørn, H., Christensena, U., & Boivinb, J. (2005). "Does Infertility Cause Marital Benefit?" An Epidemiological Study of 2250 Women and Men in Fertility Treatment. *Patient Education and Counseling, 59*(3), 244–251.

Solomon, D. H. (2016). Relational Turbulence Model. In C. R. Berger & M. E. Roloff (Eds.), *The International Encyclopaedia of Interpersonal Communication*. Hoboken, NJ: John Wiley & Sons, Inc.

Solomon, D. H., & Knobloch, L. K. (2004). A Model of Relational Turbulence: The Role of Intimacy, Relational Uncertainty, and Interference from Partners in Appraisals of Irritations. *Journal of Social and Personal Relationships, 21*(6), 795–816.

Steuber, K. R., & Solomon, D. H. (2008). Relational Uncertainty, Partner Interference, and Infertility: A Qualitative Study of Discourse within Online Forums. *Journal of Social and Personal Relationships, 25*(5), 831–855.

Steuber, K. R., & Solomon, D. H. (2012). Relational Uncertainty, Partner Interference, and Privacy Boundary Turbulence: Explaining Spousal Discrepancies in Infertility Disclosures. *Journal of Social and Personal Relationships, 29*(1), 3–27.

7

Looking Back, Moving Forward

Paulina Billett and Anne-Maree Sawyer

"And to end, I just want to say to the ladies who read this, thank you for reading and for your advice. I feel like such a dork when it comes to all of this since I've been TTC for 5 years and yet know next to nothing about the process. You all have taught me a lot and I am very grateful for all your invaluable advice and friendship!" (Joan)

In Closing

As we conclude our exploration of the experiences of those who suffer from infertility, we wish to take the time to circle back to the main issues, postulate on the challenges ahead as well as suggesting some ways forward. We have endeavoured to show through each chapter that motherhood for many women is not a certainty, but a deeply personal struggle which at times may remain unresolved. While most of the women who shared their

P. Billett (✉) • A.-M. Sawyer
La Trobe University, Melbourne, Australia
e-mail: p.billett@latorbe.edu.au; a.sawyer@latrobe.edu.au

© The Author(s) 2019
P. Billett, A.-M. Sawyer, *Infertility and Intimacy in an Online Community*,
Palgrave Macmillan Studies in Family and Intimate Life,
https://doi.org/10.1057/978-1-137-44981-8_7

stories with us eventually become mothers, their struggles were life altering. Of those who continued writing in their journals, even long after becoming mothers, it was evident that the "roller-coaster" of fertility treatments had deeply affected the way they saw themselves as women and as mothers. Many referred to their infertility journey as a nightmare and motherhood as an awakening from it. While the new journey of motherhood was seen as tough, a number of women felt that the road to motherhood could mean they would be more dedicated as mothers, and that they had reached a new level of empathy for those undergoing life struggles.

The impact of infertility, even after motherhood is achieved, shows that western constructions of femininity, which continue to be closely tied to motherhood, are damaging. In fact, as suggested in Chap. 2, the inability to achieve motherhood can lead to poor mental health outcomes and is a major contributor of depression (Newton et al. 1999). For many women, their inability to conceive was seen as a monumental failure of themselves to do something which was perceived as "natural" and the birthright of every female. For these women, the apparent betrayal of their bodies and a failure to meet expected feminine standards was undeniably devastating. These feelings were further exacerbated due to infertility remaining a largely unacknowledged issue in most societies, with fertility portrayed as a "simple" process requiring only the most casual of sexual contact for pregnancy to ensue.

The belief that pregnancy is simple is so powerful that enormous amounts of time, effort and funding are spent every year by governments around the globe on safe sex education for young people, with the aim of mitigating the "risk" of pregnancy which must "inevitably" result from intercourse. This follows into women's reproductive years, during which women go to great pains to avoid pregnancy. The possibility of infertility is not something that makes it into mainstream school curriculum or even into the fancy flyers so often found in doctors' offices; rather, it is something that couples often discover slowly after months of agonising "trying". Thus, it is unsurprising that women feel "blindsided" by their inability to easily fall pregnant and are essentially unprepared for the reality that not every couple will have a smooth road to parenthood.

The journey of infertility is inarguably a tough one, changing those who navigate it in profound ways. Most significantly, it is people's relationships that are deeply altered by this journey. Through each chapter we have engaged with different aspects of the infertility journey and its impact on relationships between the infertile individual and their (offline) family/friends, their partner, and their online friendships. We discussed the ways the women perceived themselves through their actual and imagined interactions within these relationships; and we considered the strategies the women employed to survive in what they often experienced as a hostile fertile world. Below, we turn our attention back to each of these discussions and contemplate the road ahead.

Relationships in the Infertile World

Throughout this book we suggest that infertility is a critical situation (Giddens 1979); a major kind of disruptive experience which can severely affect a woman's biography, irrevocably changing the ways in which she sees herself and conducts her everyday life. In the women's own words, we saw descriptions of how they saw themselves before and after their diagnosis with positive attributes such as "happy", "outgoing" and self-assured being used by many to describe their former "pre-infertility selves". When describing their post-diagnosis selves, most women referred to their bodies as "broken", particularly after multiple unsuccessful attempts, and labelled themselves as constantly angry, jealous and obsessed.

Time and time again we encountered posts, which discussed the experiences of infertility and the way in which these experiences had shifted their self-perceptions. Women often despaired, particularly after unsuccessful treatments, at their body's inability to do what they felt was "normal" and wondered why they were dealt this hand by destiny. Countless posts and journals described these feelings of inadequacy in great detail and often associated the failure to fall pregnant or carry to term as a loss of femininity, whether due to the effects of treatment (e.g. bloating and rapid weight gain—what women often discussed as "feeling gross") or due to their inability to achieve the ultimate feminine role—motherhood. The disruption in women's biographies was keenly felt by many and this was often given voice in journals and posts with musings of how much life had changed as well as wondering what the future held. In their respective posts, Maddison and Patricia each explain this sense of doom about the future:

I am so down right now, fourth failed cycle and now I am not sure what to do. I never thought my life would turn out this way, we had always wanted to have kids while we were young but … sometimes I sit there at night and just wonder what life will be like without children … (Maddison)

I wish I had the years on my side, but I don't and all I sit around thinking about is our potential child when he/she is 5 and we are 50! And all the young 30 year old parents that will have kids that are friends with mine and how we may never make that parent bond with others because what 30 year old would want to hang with two people in their 50's! And then I think of the child that won't have young parents who will do all that fun stuff with them that young parents can do …….and how this child's parents will be old and needing possible care before they themselves have had a chance to enjoy their lives and start lives of their own! It just never ends … (Patricia)

The dread of a radically altered future from the one they had imagined for themselves drove some women to great lengths in an attempt to understand, treat and "cure" their infertility. This occurred in two main ways: searching for information in the online world and doing all that was possible to achieve the longed for BFP.

Searching for information outside what has been provided by a treating physician has become commonplace among patients—and while we circle back to the changes this has created in the doctor-patient relationship a little later in this chapter—we wish now to turn our attention to the issues discussed in earlier sections of the book which address the effects that information seeking behaviour can have on the lives of those suffering from infertility. For many women, needing to understand and thus ensure that their treatment was as effective as possible became a self-described obsession. By their own admissions, women spent considerable time ruminating on the causes of their condition as well as searching for possible answers in traditional and alternative treatments. In a number of journal entries examined in earlier chapters, we saw that women often felt they were losing control and believed that their constant preoccupation with infertility had become an obsession that was taking over their lives (see Chaps. 4 and 6). What was highly worrisome to many was the fact that, not only was this behaviour dominating much of their waking hours, it had led in many cases to severe difficulties in couples' relationships, with several women journaling about this impact. In many of her journal entries, Patricia discussed her ever-present preoccupation with infertility and its treatment, along with the myriad stresses these persistent ruminations produced. In one such entry, Patricia stated that this behaviour was "ruining" her marriage; similarly, Mary recounted a fight with her husband in which he labelled her behaviour as "obsessive".

For these women, the labelling of their behaviour as obsessive was not only deeply enraging, but also an isolating experience. As we explored earlier in this book, negative responses towards the intense feelings aroused by the experience of infertility were seen as evidence of lack of support and understanding. The inability of their partner to feel as they did was intensely frustrating as was their lax attitude towards treatment. In one post, Caroline writes about how she feels that she and her partner "are not always on the same page" and while she feels a need to talk about their infertility experiences every day, he does not feel the same. She goes on to relate that this often leads to her "keeping it inside", resulting in intense feelings of hurt and isolation. In response, Karen and Payten replied that women on Stronger Together often experience these feelings and give advice such as "… you two should sit down and have a real heart to heart" and "… guys just think totally differently from us. It doesn't consume them like it consumes us." However, as seen in Chap. 6, men are often just as consumed by the subject of infertility as women and usually hide their feelings due to the perception that men should play supporting roles in the infertility journey. As such, many men, as reported by Hanna and Gough (2016, 2017) conceal their own fears and insecurities in order to protect their partners.

Unsurprisingly, most women sought a "couple approach" to infertility; that is, for their partner to show the same level of support and commitment (including attendance at appointments, seeking of information and willingness to try alternative therapies) in the conception of a child, as they themselves had invested. However, the intense focus on the female body through ART treatment coupled with the close association of femininity and motherhood, mean that many women will continue to feel alone on this journey. In fact, the close link between motherhood and femininity has produced a situation in which women see their infertility as a tragedy while men, whose role as fathers is not as closely tied to masculinity, do not. As such, according to the women's accounts, and at least on the surface, most men did not suffer from the same level of biographical disruption which women experienced through the potential loss of parenthood. Men were often reported as finding the experience of infertility difficult due to the association of masculinity and male fertility. As suggested by Hanna and Gough (2016, 2017), men were highly preoccupied with how infertility affected their virility, often discussing similar issues as the women, but not in terms of fatherhood—rather, as an intense preoccupation with the societal stigma attached to the perceived "lack of capacity" ascribed to infertile men.

As discussed in some depth in Chap. 6, men were often anxious about being labelled "infertile". For these men, simple requests to undertake alternative treatments, take vitamins or even collect prescriptions were sources of anxiety. While masculinity is not closely tied to fatherhood, it is intimately linked to sexual performance. Thus, for male partners to run the risk of being "discovered" or even presumed to be an underperforming male was something many women seemed determined to avoid. In fact, many women felt it their responsibility to protect their partner from potential scrutiny. Often couched in terms of care for their partner and thus their relationship, the women of Stronger Together took great pains to shield their partners from the realities of the journey by ensuring that they took responsibility for the bulk of the treatment. This entailed "normalising" their journey by manufacturing an illusion of spontaneity around sexual activity, acting as a protector against the distress of male factor, and acting as a buffer against the stresses and demands of fertility treatment.

As we saw in Chap. 6, women frequently took over responsibility during treatment; whether it was in protecting their partners from the realities of the journey or simply ensuring that they had done everything in their power to achieve pregnancy or carry to term. However, the pressure to do everything was frequently overwhelming and few women coped from cycle to cycle with the intense demands. As we have seen through the women's accounts, members of Stronger Together needed to deal with the uncertainty of the infertility journey. Often referred to as the "roller-coaster", this journey is punctuated by thrilling highs (usually in the way of hope after treatment or with the announcement of a BFP) and soul crushing lows when treatment did not work or a pregnancy was lost. Most of those who shared their journeys with us did not fall pregnant within the first two cycles, but instead took years trying to concieve, perhaps considered adoption, or simply "waited" to decide how to harness their retreating dreams of motherhood. This meant that the hopefulness which was so typically part of the early phases of journey had by the conclusion of our research project lost much of its promise for many of these women. In these situations, supportive advice to "stay positive" was frequently encouraged by OSG participants; engaging in positive thinking, even against the odds, seemed to be the main currency of exchange, advice and support in Stronger Together (see Chap. 4).

As we described in Chap. 4, the need to maintain a positive and hopeful outlook was at times a heavy burden, particularly for those confronted by endless treatment cycles, or those who after miscarriage needed to begin all over once again. Many of those who commenced treatment were already exhausted by the repeated failures they had experienced as, according to many of the women's stories, the decision to try fertility treatment had not been made lightly but had been taken after long periods of testing and attempts to achieve pregnancy "naturally". For these women, fertility specialists represented their last chance at motherhood. The hope that fertility treatment would finally and quickly deliver a precious baby was largely underpinned by the fantasy, sold by fertility clinics, suggesting that pregnancy will ensue almost immediately after ART treatment. However, as the years rolled on and the women did not achieve pregnancy or carry to term, the realities and demands of fertility treatment soon took their toll.

Many found it increasingly difficult to rely on hope and positive thinking to maintain the arduous demands of the infertility journey and those further along the journey increasingly doubted the possibilities of success and despaired at this realisation (e.g. see Chap. 4). When their capacities to conform to the discourse of positive thinking failed, others in the online support group provided a fountain of new strength through words of encouragement. In posts and messages, women were encouraged by others to "keep going", with women often alluding to others' successes as "evidence" of the fulfilment of the promises made by doctors at the beginning of their journeys. This was enough for many to re-engage in the process of positive thinking. Elisabeth discusses this in one of her journals:

> I've had a bit of a negative attitude recently, having little panics that it's just never going to happen. I know, logically, that the odds are in favour of me eventually getting pregnant, but it's hard to keep telling yourself that as the months pass. Overall, though, my stress has gone down significantly while on this break, and I've kept very busy with friends and the holidays, but whether it's hormones or just the reality check that AF brings, this week's just been a little tough. It's nice to have this little refuge, where I can come and read success stories to feel inspired, or vent my frustrations. Thank you ST!

We believe that this constant reassurance is problematic, as women who are too exhausted to continue treatment would repeatedly find these reassurances seductive enough to spur them on without any real evaluation of whether they should in fact continue. What is more, these reassurances coupled with the unrealistic picture painted by fertility clinics further motivated others to push on. As a result, the belief that pregnancy is just around the corner sets up women to blame themselves for resulting BFNs and miscarriages, which they frequently feel is the result of their having missed some vital step rather than seeing it as the most likely result of ART treatments' low success rates. In the light of this, we believe that a more accurate portrayal of pregnancy needs to be made, one that not only deals with the realities of infertility, but also sees regulation of the ART market. In particular, we believe this needs to occur in relation to the claims on success which clinics are able to make. This we feel is essential to improving sufferers' expectations of their treatment and their long-term wellbeing.

The emotional roller-coaster of high expectations of success, and repeated experiences of failure, was further exacerbated by episodes of having to deal, sometimes in very intimate ways, with others who could "easily" conceive. As we have described throughout this book, infertility is an issue, which many find difficult to talk about, and it is a topic about which most seem to prefer to remain silent. Misconceptions about infertility still abound, and couples frequently feel a deep sense of shame at their inability to conceive or carry a pregnancy to term. The stigma surrounding infertility, including the belief that infertility must be the cause of promiscuity (particularly on the women's part), women have "left it too late", the couple is just "not meant" to have children or simply that they are "wound too tight" and that conception will happen if they just "relax" or adopt. This type of unhelpful advice or insensitive comments often came from the closest of quarters, with many of the women reporting their family (particularly their mothers) and closest friends as the main antagonists (for an indepth discussion see Chap. 5). For the women who shared their journeys with us, the inability of those closest to them to "take their role" as infertility sufferers, was a source of great frustration and insensitive comments or ill-informed opinions were seen as further evidence of how truly alone they were on their IF journey.

In line with our findings, it is our belief that the silence surrounding infertility is highly damaging for suffers. As we have seen, relationships can be severely affected by the inability of others to appreciate the wide-reaching impact of infertility on an individual; we believe this inability to take the sufferer's role is largely the product of the lack of information and education currently available on this condition. Presently there are no government campaigns (at least that we are aware of) that promote an even basic understanding of this condition. In fact, it could be argued that it has been the exact opposite. In several countries around the globe, governments have used popular opinion and myths surrounding infertility to pass laws banning certain ART practices (e.g. surrogacy) or lower the funding which couples receive for treatment cycles (see Introduction for some of these debates). These changes have been made without evaluating the impact such discourse can have on sufferers or how they perpetuate incorrect notions of infertility. As such, we, in line with peak bodies such as ACCESS and RESOLVE, suggest that community discussion and education of the prevalence and impact of infertility is urgently needed. We believe this to be particularly true considering the suggestion made by peak bodies such as the United Nations that infertility is a growing issue among global communities. While we do not foresee a change in the very near future, our hope is that as more couples access these services, a concerted effort will be made to bring better community understanding of this condition.

Announcement of pregnancies and births were always hard for the women of Stronger Together. For many, the emotions which these announcements generated were a source of much confusion as happiness for the new parents mingled with sadness for their own childless situation. The women of Stronger Together often gave voice to these sentiments in the form of "venting". Discussions in journals and posts about new pregnancy announcements were often accompanied by intense feelings of jealousy, anger and confusion. Posts and journals provided a place for introspection as well as the opportunity to seek reassurance from others that these feelings were in fact "normal" (for example, see Chaps. 5 and 6). The countless journals we encountered which sought advice on how to deal with this situation, almost always received high levels of response. These responses were often accompanied by calls to not lose hope as "your turn is next".

The impact of infertility on offline relationships also crossed into the virtual world through social media. We often encountered posts and journal entries from women who discussed the impact of technology on already destabilised relationships. In an especially poignant entry in Elisabeth's journal (discussed in Chap. 5), she wonders "why I torture myself" by going "onto Facebook" and learning of others' pregnancies and births: "I really should just block everyone who has small children. I can't handle seeing the pictures without bawling, but I look anyway. I feel horrible that I can't just be happy for them without feeling so sad for myself."

Lilly echoed this in her journal:

> Well my nephew's GF just keeps putting up baby crap CONSTANTLY on FB and I can't take it anymore! She even tagged me in one picture! Wish I could have punched her!!! So every time it happens I say to myself, I'm going to block her and I obviously never do … and then I spend hours looking at her baby pictures … sick or what!

Blocking friends on social media was seen by many as a viable way in which to manage this uncomfortable situation, however, as can be seen by these excerpts, the women often did not take this step. The continual engagement in what many described as agony was partly related to the fear of discovery, that is of their friends and relations finding out that they had been blocked, but it was also a way in which to maintain a semblance of control over their wayward emotions, by simply "dealing" with the emotional onslaught of photographs of babies and sonograms. In this way, the fertile world was extended for the women of Stronger Together into their homes and daily lives, further exacerbating the women's intense feelings of isolation. For these women, no place is safe, and fertility is everywhere but in their own wombs.

While the online world often buffeted the women's emotions, it also provided an important refuge. As we have seen, relationships in the infertile world are highly complicated and need to be carefully negotiated. Online support groups such as Stronger Together provided uncomplicated relationships based on the experiences of being infertile; a place where understanding and support is guaranteed.

A Refuge from the Storm: Online Support Groups

The rise of the internet in the 1990s, with the invention of the world wide web by Tim Berners-Lee, saw the creation of a unique space in which individuals were no longer bound by geography in their support group participation. Suddenly, individuals could access help for any number of conditions from the comfort of their own homes. This was an important development for individuals suffering from conditions with life altering, often irremediable and highly stigmatising consequences such as infertility. The birth of OSGs afforded companionship, understanding and 24/7 support, while the anonymity of the online world ensured that individuals could openly share their experiences without fear of being recognised by others. OSGs such as Stronger Together play an essential role in the lives of infertile women. The rise of the OSG has radically altered the ways individuals approach treatment and seek advice and support (Mo and Coulson 2014, p. 984). As we have seen throughout this book, the fertile world can be perilous for those who feel that they do not belong to it. One of the strategies used to gain a sense of belonging has been in finding support in OSGs such as Stronger Together, which affords its members support, intimacy and understanding. The role of OSGs is becoming ever more important as the reach of the internet expands further every day and now provides a support group for almost every conceivable issue/illness/condition. For those suffering from fertility issues, these online support groups are a boon; not only are individuals able to pick and choose between groups to suit their own personality, but they are no longer bound by distance or precluded from attending due to embarrassment.

Through our time in Stronger Together, we saw countless posts which aimed to introduce new members to the community. These new members almost always expressed relief at having found a place where not only did they feel welcome, but also could find support, companionship and most importantly, information. In her post, Rita, after describing what the last three years of trying and testing had been like, stated that she was looking for "some support and encouragement that all will be well …" She received the encouragement and support she so craved, with respondents to this thread, replying as follows:

Loren: "… there are people like you out there who totally understand what you are going through!"
Carrie: "… This is a wonderful place of supportive and caring women …"
Tina: "… I am here for you. WE are all going through it together …"
Becky: "I have found incredible support and advice here … you know you are not alone …"

Support such as this is important, as the stigma attached to the infertility journey can at times stop women from seeking support from offline friends and family. As we have discussed previously, for these women, having others who could understand their unique position was incredibly important and Stronger Together allowed them to belong to a community of likeminded others. It also allowed them to make sense of their journey by providing a place in which to give expression to the traumatic feelings encountered on the journey without the fear of feeling judged. For these women, Stronger Together was an oasis, where their feelings, even the most negative, were validated, and their "scripts" rewritten in reflection with, and alongside, those of other members.

Aside from the ability to make new friends and belong to a community who understood their unique challenges, Stronger Together provided an opportunity for women to gain informational assistance (Tanis 2007) in the form of information on treatment options. As we explored in Chap. 2 and again in Chap. 3, a large percentage of posts was dedicated to asking others about their experiences of traditional and alternative treatments, as well as double-checking on the appropriateness of the treatments individuals were currently receiving. As we discussed in Chap. 3, many women became disheartened with the detachment displayed by professional medical staff, and often discussed this vexation with others on Stronger Together. As was presented in earlier sections, responses encouraging the questioning of medical expertise were often encountered and the longer participants remained in the group, the more likely it was for them to shift from passive recipient of treatment to well-informed, active patient, not afraid to challenge medical teams in their search for parenthood. This shift in the patient/doctor relationship has meant that clinics and doctors have had to rethink their approach to their relationships with their patients as women become more demanding and less tolerant of what they perceive as substandard or "heartless" treatment of their condition. Unsurprisingly, fertility clinics can now be found to include wording suggesting a caring and companionate approach, which features individualised and patient-centred treatment (for some examples of this see the websites of IVF Australia, Monash IVF, The fertility institutes, Life IVF centre, Bourne Hall Fertility Clinic, The Agora Gynaecology & Fertility Centre). However, whether these promises are delivered remains unclear. If the experiences related in Stronger Together are representative of most women's encounters with fertility treatment, this is certainly not the case. Yet, it is hoped that as patients become increasingly engaged and insist on a more empathic form of care, it will help to drive a change in culture.

Infertility OSGs and Implications for Professional Therapeutic Practice

The proliferation of such open-access OSGs as Stronger Together presents a source of very useful material for therapists and counsellors working with women or couples who are infertile. These sites offer unfettered access into the very particular emotional worlds of women suffering from infertility, thus enabling helping professionals to "more fully understand the emotional and informational needs" of this group and thereby "improve the level of psychosocial support offered to [them]" (Malik and Coulson 2008b, p. 112). As we have shown in the foregoing chapters, Stronger Together illuminated the minutiae of the women's daily concerns as they navigated their individual IF journeys—what to eat, how to exercise and what to think, all in an effort to achieve a BFP. These micro-details demonstrate the extent to which a host of disciplinary practices are woven into their everyday lives, producing additional stresses and sources of self-blame beyond the shame of infertility itself. Through perusing such sites, one may also discern the women's sense-making processes, specifically the narrative resources they use to frame their own and fellow members' experiences of the distress and failure that characterises the roller-coaster ride of infertility. For such sympathy workers as therapists, counsellors, and nurses, these sites offer a means of extending one's sympathies by learning more about the firsthand experiences of this very poorly understood condition, from the perspectives of the sufferers themselves.

Our study has elucidated the dominant narratives that guided the online interactions of Stronger Together members. These findings are useful in demonstrating to helping professionals the way in which the women are often caught between the promises of biotechnology, and the individualising forces of positive thinking and biopolitics. A key function of therapeutic practice is to illuminate the socio-cultural narratives in which individuals participate (Holmes 2016; Illouz 2008) to heighten their consciousness of the social arrangements and power relations that shape their personal experiences. Where helpful, therapists and counsellors may collaborate with women to shine a light on the broader context of infertility, namely the multi-billion dollar fertility treatment industry, the apparent misinformation about success rates of live births following ART, and the lack of support available for women to decide when to "stop" treatment (ABC TV 2016; Greil et al. 2011; Leigh 2016). In some situations, recognition of these broader socio-cultural factors may be therapeutic in itself.

With reference to the "sociological imagination" (Wright Mills 1959), personal troubles are always located in particular times and places. People's stories are thus works of history, social structure and biography. Attention to "the social" in personal stories "can be interpreted for the ways it supports and/or undermines larger systems of domination" (Riessman 2001, p. 75). In considering women's identity construction in the context of infertility, therapists might facilitate women's therapeutic journeys by considering the breadth of the "the social": the women's own resources for dealing with infertility, including their involvement in an OSG; the reactions of significant others; the IF industry; and, the quality of their relationships with healthcare professionals. Working with this big picture view in a supportive, therapeutic setting may facilitate the process of "working through": deconstructing these social arrangements to show their shaping influences on individual lives. This approach could also illuminate the lack of (coherent) culturally prescribed narratives available to guide women in living beyond multiple failed IVF attempts (Leigh 2016). In so doing, it may show the ambiguous and disenfranchised nature of grief associated with infertility (Doka 1989, 2002), thus providing explanatory insights into the jarring experiences of emotional entrapment (see Chap. 5).

Time and again, our study revealed the usefulness of OSG participation to women in the midst of their IF journeys, particularly the empowering and supportive effects of participation (Barak et al. 2008; Bartlett and Coulson 2011). Thus, therapists and counsellors have a role in encouraging such participation in conjunction with their face-to-face therapies, but only when appropriate. We fully acknowledge that, for some women, having to encounter entreaties to "stay positive", for example, are counterproductive—particularly when struggling with a decision to end treatment (see Kate's post in Chap. 4).

Researching into the Future

The impact of infertility treatment on women's sense of identity is not something that can be settled by a single study but should be a work in progress. As described by our participants, the stigma of fertility treatment never fully disappears, and some women experience a sense of dissonance well after they have successfully given birth to their children. For this reason, we believe an examination into how women negotiate life after fertility treatment is essential, in order to more fully understand the long-term impact of fertility treatment. We also suggest that more research be undertaken on the changes couples experience after fertility treatment, especially as the realities of parenthood sink in. Finally, we suggest that the largely untold stories of women childless not by choice are examined. This we feel is essential, as the myth of fertility treatment is predicated on successful conception and delivery of a much-wanted child. For the most part, women who have been unsuccessful in their pursuit of motherhood slip away from sites such as Stronger Together once they have given up all hope of becoming mothers. However, searches for comparable sites which cater for women childless not by choice are very few, suggesting that this may be a very lonely part of the journey (Leigh 2016). As a result, we urge that more research be undertaken on this stage of the infertility roller-coaster in order to ensure that all aspects of the infertility journey are understood.

Conclusion

In concluding this book, we would like to thank the brave women of Stronger Together for sharing their stories with us. What we have seen is that infertility is a life altering experience, one that even years later can affect how women see themselves. Infertility is a condition which is only set to increase over the coming years. If projections from the United Nations are right, by 2050, eight of the largest countries will have below birth rate replacement levels. For many, the road to parenthood will be easier, requiring little if any assistance to form a family. However, for others, this may not be the case and increasing numbers of couples will require the help of ART.

However, even while the numbers are set to increase, our discussions around fertility continue to be based on the myth of simple pregnancy. It is hoped that as more couples enter the uncertain road of the infertility journey, the much-needed systemic change occurs, and that the sheer volume of voices finally opens discussion on the realities facing infertile couples.

In the future, the role which OSGs play will continue to grow, as individuals look for the kind of support so obviously lacking in their offline relationships. Places such as Stronger Together will continue as refuges from the storm and will harbour the stories of personal struggle for self-acceptance, which the infertility journey arouses. OSGs will continue to be places where women can, at least for a time, sidestep the minefield laden territory of relationships with others in the "fertile world" and continue to find strength for their journey to possible motherhood.

References

Australian Broadcasting Commission ABC TV. (2016). The Baby Business. *Four Corners* (Broadcast May-30). Retrieved from http://www.abc.net.au/4corners/stories/2016/05/30/4469652.htm.

Barak, A., Boniel-Nissim, M., & Suler, J. (2008). Fostering Empowerment in Online Support Groups. *Computers in Human Behavior, 24*(5), 1867–1883.

Bartlett, Y. K., & Coulson, N. S. (2011). An Investigation into the Empowerment Effects of Using Online Support Groups and How This Affects Health Professional/Patient Communication. *Patient Education and Counseling, 83*(1), 113–119.

Doka, K. J. (1989). *Disenfranchised Grief: Recognizing Hidden Sorrow*. Lexington: Lexington Books.

Doka, K. J. (2002). *Disenfranchised Grief: New Directions, Challenges and Strategies for Practice*. Champaign, IL: Research Press.

Giddens, A. (1979). *Central Problems in Social Theory*. London: Macmillan.

Greil, A., McQuillan, J., & Slauson-Blevins, K. (2011). The Social Construction of Infertility. *Sociology Compass, 5*(8), 736–746.

Hanna, E., & Gough, B. (2016). Emoting Infertility Online: A Qualitative Analysis of Men's Forum Posts. *Health, 20*(4), 363–382.

Hanna, E., & Gough, B. (2017). Men's Accounts of Infertility Within Their Intimate Partner Relationships: An Analysis of Online Forum Discussions. *Journal of Reproductive and Infant Psychology, 35*(2), 150–158.

Holmes, K. (2016). Talking About Mental Illness: Life Histories and Mental Health in Modern Australia. *Australian Historical Studies, 47*(1), 25–40.

Illouz, E. (2008). *Saving the Modern Soul: Therapy, Emotions, and the Culture of Self-Help.* Berkeley, CA: University of California Press.

Leigh, J. (2016). *Avalanche: A Love Story.* Melbourne: Penguin Group Australia.

Malik, S. H., & Coulson, N. S. (2008a). Computer-Mediated Infertility Support Groups: An Exploratory Study of Online Experiences. *Patient Education and Counseling, 73*(1), 105–113.

Malik, S. H., & Coulson, N. S. (2008b). The Male Experience of Infertility: A Thematic Analysis of an Online Infertility Support Group Bulletin Board. *Journal of Reproductive and infant psychology, 26*(1), 18–30.

Mo, P. K. H., & Coulson, N. S. (2014). Are Online Support Groups Always Beneficial? A Qualitative Exploration of the Empowering and Disempowering Processes of Participation Within HIV/AIDS-Related Online Support Groups. *International Journal of Nursing Studies, 51*(7), 983–993.

Newton, C. R., Sherrad, W., & Glavac, I. (1999). The Fertility Problem Inventory: Measuring Perceived Fertility Related Stress. *Fertility and Sterility, 72*(1), 54–62.

Riessman, C. K. (2001). Personal Troubles as Social Issues: A Narrative of Infertility in Context. In I. Shaw & N. Gould (Eds.), *Qualitative Research in Social Work* (pp. 73–83). London: Sage.

Tanis, M. (2007). Online Social Support Groups. In A. N. Joinson, K. Y. A. McKenna, T. Postmes, & U.-D. Reips (Eds.), *The Oxford Handbook of Internet Psychology* (pp. 139–153). Oxford: Oxford University Press.

Wright Mills, C. (1959). *The Sociological Imagination.* Oxford: Oxford University Press.

Appendix A: Codes Used in Analysis of Journals and Posts

Avoidance
Avoidance—of others
Avoidance—of situations
Cessation of treatment
Cessation of treatment—desire to
Cessation of treatment—due to medical issue
Cessation of treatment—fear of
Cessation of treatment—taking time off
Changes to biography
Changes to lifestyle
Changes to lifestyle—negative
Changes to lifestyle—positive
Children
Children—future-children
Children—living
Children—wanting
Children—miscarriage or stillbirth
Community
Community—offline
Community—offline—positive
Community—offline—negative experience
Community online

© The Author(s) 2019
P. Billett, A.-M. Sawyer, *Infertility and Intimacy in an Online Community*,
Palgrave Macmillan Studies in Family and Intimate Life,
https://doi.org/10.1057/978-1-137-44981-8

Community online—positive experience
Community online—negative experience
Couple relationship
Couple relationship—bad
Couple relationship—deteriorating
Couple relationship—good
Couple relationship—improving
Husband or partner
Co-worker
Dealing with
Dealing with—other people's ultrasounds
Dealing with—pregnancy announcement
Dealing with—pregnant woman
Difference in IF experience
Emotion management—strategies (e.g. reading success stories to boost mood,
   trying not to be bitter about others, thinking positively)
Ethical questions
Poor parenting
Factor
Factor—Female
Factor—Male
Factor—Unexplained
Failure
Failure—of relationship
Failure—of self
Failure—of treatment
Failure—of work
Faith
Faith—turn to
Faith—decrease
Faith—increase
Father
Feelings
Feeling—anger, resentment
Feeling—anger or resentment toward ex-partner
Feeling—anger, resentment toward family
Feeling—anger, resentment toward friends
Feeling—anger, resentment toward God
Feeling—anger, resentment toward life
Feeling—anger, resentment toward colleague(s)
Feeling—anger, resentment toward doctor
Feeling—apprehension
Feeling—confusion
Feeling—hurt
Feeling—isolation

Feeling—joy
Feelings—joy—good response
Feelings—joy—natural pregnancy
Feelings—joy—other
Feelings—joy—adoption
Feelings—joy—successful treatment
Feeling—positive
Feeling—broken
Feeling—frustration
Feelings—anxiety
Feelings—disappointment
Feelings—excitement
Feelings—fear
Fear of—childlessness not by choice
Fear of—unsuccessful treatment
Feelings—guilt
Feelings—hope
Feelings—have hope
Feelings—lacking or losing hope
Feelings—longing
Feelings—relief
Feelings—sadness
Feelings—stressed
Female
Financial pressure
First time user
First time user—seeking information
First time user—seeking support
Friends
Friend—as support
Friend—cause of sadness
Friends—avoidance of
Frenemy
Identity crisis
Impact of infertility
Information
Information—seeking
Information seeking—how to deal with other
Information seeking—how to deal with situation
Information seeking—medical
Information seeking—sexual
Information giving
Information giving
Information giving—how to deal with other
Information giving—medical

Information giving—sexual
Injustice of infertility (why is it happening to me?)
Miscarriage due to
Blighted ovum
Early miscarriage (less than 12 weeks)
Ectopic
Late miscarriage (over 12 weeks)
Misunderstood by
colleague(s)
Doctor
Family
Friends
Mother
Mother—problem
Mother—support
Mother in law
Mother in law—support
Mother in law—problem
Motherhood
Motherhood—will be a good mother
Motherhood—adoption
Motherhood—angel baby
Motherhood—childless
Motherhood—feeling less
Motherhood—foster care
Motherhood—meaning
Pregnant other
Relationships
Good relationships
Relationship—good—colleagues
Relationship—good—doctor
Relationship—good—family
Relationship—good—friends
Relationship—improving relationships
Relationship—improving—family
Relationship—improving relationship—colleagues
Relationship—improving relationship—doctor
Relationship—improving relationship—friends
Relationship—bad
Relationship—bad—family
Relationship—bad with friends
Relationship—bad—doctor
Relationship—bad—colleague(s)
Relationships—deteriorating
Relationships—deteriorating—doctor

Relationships—deteriorating—friends
Relationships—deteriorating colleagues
Relationships—deteriorating—family
Self-care
Self-improvement
Working on the self/setting goals
Self-image
Self-image—less of a woman
Self-image—negative
Self-image—positive
Self-image—survivor
Self-surveillance (in terms of working on the self, eating healthy foods)
Self-monitoring
Sex
Sex—description of
Sex—issues with
Sex—seeking advice
Sibling
Sibling—problem
Sibling—support
Sick role
Societal perceptions
Negative societal perceptions
Positive societal perceptions
Support
Support—lacking
Support—having
Treatment—length
Treatment
Treatment—IVF
Treatment—Clomid
Treatment—FET
Treatment—ICSI
Treatment—IUI
Treatment—natural therapy
Treatment—poor medical
Treatment—questioning medical
Treatment—impact of
Length of treatment
Negative impact of treatment
Positive impact of treatment
Trolls
Trust in the universe
Unwanted advice
Use of site

Use of site—grief
Use of site—musing
Use of site—sharing background
Use of site—sharing change in lifestyle
Use of site—sharing disappointment
Use of site—sharing fears
Use of site—sharing frustration
Use of site—sharing medical
Use of site—sharing sadness
Use of site—thanking others
Use of site—venting
Use of site—sharing excitement
Use of site—sharing hope
Use of site—sharing joy
Work

Appendix B: Common Abbreviations Used on Stronger Together Site

2ww	Two Week Wait (Luteal Phase—14 days after ovulation)

A

AF	Aunt Flo, menstruation, period
AFNW	Aunt Flo Not Wanted
AH	Assisted Hatching
AI	Artificial Insemination
ANA	Anti-Nuclear Antibodies
ART	Assisted Reproductive Technology

B

Baby Dust	Good wishes for getting pregnant
BBT	Basal Body Temperature
BCP	Birth Control Pills
BD	Baby Dance, Sex
BETA	Blood test for PG
BF	Best Friend or Boy Friend
BFN	Big Fat Negative (Pregnancy Tests)
BFP	Big Fat Positive (Pregnancy Test)
BW	Blood work

© The Author(s) 2019   **191**
P. Billett, A.-M. Sawyer, *Infertility and Intimacy in an Online Community*,
Palgrave Macmillan Studies in Family and Intimate Life,
https://doi.org/10.1057/978-1-137-44981-8

C

CB	Cycle Buddy—Same cycle day as you!
CCCT	Clomiphene Citrate Challenge Test (Clomid Challenge)
CD	Cycle Day
CM	Cervical Mucus CF Cervical Fluid
CP	Cervical Position

D

DB	Dear Boyfriend
D&C	Dilation & Curettage
DD	Dear Daughter
DE	Donor Eggs
DH	Dear Husband
DI	Donor Insemination
Do	Diagnosis
DP	Dancing Partner (Dancing refers to intercourse); spouse, or significant other
DPO	Days Past Ovulation
DS	Dear Son
DT	Day Transfer

E

E2	Estradiol
EB	Endometrial Biopsy
EDD	Estimated Due Date
Endo	Endometriosis
EP	Ectopic Pregnancy
EPT	Early Pregnancy Test
ER	Egg Retrieval
ET	Embryo Transfer
EWCM	Egg-White Cervical Mucus

F

FB	Follicular Phase
FET	Frozen Embryo Transfer
FSH	Follicle Stimulating Hormone

G

GP	General Practitioner

H

H&H	Happy and Healthy
HCG	Human Chronic Gonadotropin—detected in HPTs
HPT	Home Pregnancy Test
HSG	Hysterosalpingogram—x-ray
HX	History

I

IF	Infertility
IUI	Intrauterine Insemination
IVF	In Vitro Fertilisation

L

LAP	Laparoscopy
LH	Luteinizing Hormone—detected in OPK's
LMC	Last Menstrual Cycle
LP	Luteal Phase, days between ov & AF
LPD	Luteal Phase Defect

M

M/C	Miscarriage
MF	Male Factor

N

NP	Nurse Practitioner

O

O/OV	Ovulation
OB/GYN	Obstetrician/Gynaecologist
OPK	Ovulation Predictor Kit

P

PCOS	Polycystic Ovarian Syndrome
PG	Pregnancy, pregnant
PI	Primary Infertility
PNV	Prenatal Vitamin
POAS	Pee on a Stick—pregnancy test
PTS	Pregnancy Test Strip

R

RE	Reproductive Endocrinologists—doctor who specialises in fertility problems
RSN	Real soon now
Rx	Prescription

S

SA	Semen Analysis
SI	Secondary Infertility
SO	Significant Other
STIM	Stimulating Drugs

T

TMI	Too Much Information
TR	Tubal Reversal
TTC	Trying to Conceive
Tx	Treatment

U

U/S	Ultrasound

References

Abbey, A., Andrews, F. M., & Halman, J. L. (1991). Gender Roles in Responses to Infertility. *Psychology of Women Quarterly, 15*(2), 295–316.

Abbey, A., Andrews, F. M., & Halman, J. L. (1995). Provision and Receipt of Social Support and Disregard: What Is Their Impact on the Marital Life Quality of Infertile and Fertile Couples? *Journal of Personality and Social Psychology, 68*(3), 455–469.

Acker, J., Barry, K., & Joke, E. (1983). Objectivity and Truth: Problems in Doing Feminist Research. *Women's Studies International Forum, 6*(4), 423–435.

Australian Broadcasting Commission ABC TV. (2016). The Baby Business. *Four Corners* (Broadcast May-30). Retrieved from http://www.abc.net.au/4corners/stories/2016/05/30/4469652.htm.

Barak, A., & Dolev-Cohen, M. (2006). Does Activity Level in Online Support Groups for Distressed Adolescents Determine Emotional Relief. *Counselling and Psychotherapy Research, 6*(3), 186–190.

Barak, A., Boniel-Nissim, M., & Suler, J. (2008). Fostering Empowerment in Online Support Groups. *Computers in Human Behavior, 24*(5), 1867–1883.

© The Author(s) 2019
P. Billett, A.-M. Sawyer, *Infertility and Intimacy in an Online Community*,
Palgrave Macmillan Studies in Family and Intimate Life,
https://doi.org/10.1057/978-1-137-44981-8

Bartlett, Y. K., & Coulson, N. S. (2011). An Investigation into the Empowerment Effects of Using Online Support Groups and How This Affects Health Professional/Patient Communication. *Patient Education and Counseling, 83*(1), 113–119.

Bauman, Z. (2003). *Liquid Love: On the Frailty of Human Bonds.* Cambridge: Polity Press.

Beck, U. (1992). *Risk Society: Towards a New Modernity.* Newbury Park: Sage.

Beck, U., & Beck-Gernsheim, E. (1995). *The Normal Chaos of Love.* Oxford: Polity Press.

Beck, U., & Beck-Gernsheim, E. (2002). *Individualization: Institutionalized Individualism and Its Social and Political Consequences.* London; Thousand Oaks, CA: Sage.

Bernard, J. (1975). *Mothers, Women and Wives.* New York: Aldine Publishing Company.

Blackshaw, T. (2010). *Key Concepts in Community Studies.* London: Sage Publications.

Boyce, A. K. (2013). Protecting the Voiceless: Rights of the Child in Transnational Surrogacy Agreements. *Suffolk Transnational Law Review, 36*(3), 650–670.

Brezina, P., & Zhao, Y. (2012). The Ethical, Legal, and Social Issues Impacted by Modern Assisted Reproductive Technologies. *Obstetrics and Gynecology International,* Article ID 686253, 1–7.

Broom, A. (2009). Intuition, Subjectivity and Le bricoleur: Cancer Patients' Accounts of Negotiating a Plurality of Therapeutic Options. *Qualitative Health Research, 19*(8), 1050–1059.

Broom, A., & Tovey, P. (2007). Therapeutic Pluralism? Evidence, Power and Legitimacy in UK Cancer Services. *Sociology of Health & Illness, 29*(3), 551–569.

Brown, G. W., & Harris, T. (1978). *Social Origins of Depression: A Study of Psychiatric Disorders in Women.* Tavistock: London.

Brownlie, J. (2014). *Ordinary Relationships: A Sociological Study of Emotions, Reflexivity and Culture.* London: Palgrave Macmillan.

Bruner, J. (1987). Life as Narrative. *Social Research, 54*(1), 11–32.

Bury, M. (1982). Chronic Illness as Biographical Disruption. *Sociology of Health & Illness, 4*(2), 167–182.

Busfield, J. (2011). *Mental Illness.* Cambridge: Polity Press.

Cacioppo, J. T., & Patrick, W. (2008). *Loneliness: Human Nature and the Need for Social Connection.* New York: Norton.

Campos-Castillo, C., & Hitlin, S. (2013). Copresence: Revisiting a Building Block for Social Interaction Theories. *Sociological Theory, 31*(2), 168–192.

Carmeli, S., & Birenbaum-Carmeli, D. (1994). The Predicament of Masculinity: Towards Understanding the Male's Experience of Infertility Treatments. *Sex Roles, 30*(9–10), 663–677.

Castells, M. (2001). *The Internet Galaxy: Reflections on the Internet, Business and Society*. New York: Oxford University Press.

Chachamovich, R. L., Chachamovich, J. E., Ezer, H., Fleck, M. P., Knauth, D. R., & Pandolfi Passos, E. (2010). Agreement on Perceptions of Quality of Life in Couples Dealing with Infertility. *Journal of Obstetric, Gynecologic, & Neonatal Nursing, 39*(5), 557–565.

Chambers, D. (2006). *New Social Ties: Contemporary Connections in a Fragmented Society*. Houndmills; New York: Palgrave Macmillan.

Chambers, D. (2013). *Social Media and Personal Relationships: Online Intimacies and Personal Friendships*. Basingstoke: Palgrave Macmillan.

Chase, E., & Walker, R. (2012). The Co-Construction of Shame in the Context of Poverty: Beyond a Threat to the Social Bond. *Sociology, 47*(4), 739–754.

Chung, J. E. (2013). Social Interaction in Online Support Groups: Preference for Online Social Interaction Over Offline Social Interaction. *Computers in Human Behavior, 29*(4), 1408–1414.

Clarke, C. (1997). *Misery and Company: Sympathy in Everyday Life*. Chicago: University of Chicago Press.

Cobb, S. (1976). Social Support as a Moderator of Life Stress. *Psychosomatic Medicine, 38*(5), 300–314.

Cohen, S., & Wills, T. A. (1985). Stress, Social Support and the Buffering Hypothesis. *Psychological Bulletin, 98*(2), 310–357.

Collin, P., Metcalf, A., Stephens-Reicher, J., et al. (2011). ReachOut.com: The Role of an Online Service for Promoting Help Seeking in Young People. *Advances in Mental Health, 10*(1), 39–51.

Collins, R. (2004). *Interaction Ritual Chains*. Princeton, NJ: Princeton University Press.

Coontz, S. (2004). The World Historical Transformation of Marriage. *Journal of Marriage and Family, 66*(4), 974–979.

Crawshaw, P. (2012). Governing at a Distance: Social Marketing and the Bio(Politics) of Responsibility. *Social Science & Medicine, 75*, 200–2007.

Creswell, J. (2013). *Qualitative Inquiry & Research Design: Choosing Among Five Approaches*. Thousand Oaks: Sage.

Davis, J. (2000). Accounts of False Memory Syndrome: Parents, "Retractors", and the Role of Institutions in Account Making. *Qualitative Sociology, 23*(1), 29–56.

Davison, K. P., Pennebaker, J. W., & Dickerson, S. S. (2000). Who Talks? The Social Psychology of Illness Support Groups. *American Psychologist, 55*(2), 205–217.

Denny, E. (1994). Liberation or Oppression? Radical Feminism and In Vitro Fertilisation. *Sociology of Health & Illness, 16*(1), 62–80.

Deonandan, R., Green, S., & van Beinum, A. (2012). Ethical Concerns for Maternal Surrogacy and Reproductive Tourism. *Journal of Medical Ethics, 38*(12), 742–745.

Dermott, E., & Seymour, J. (2011). Developing "Displaying Families": A Possibility for the Future of the Sociology of Personal Life. In E. Dermott & J. Seymour (Eds.), *Displaying Families: A New Concept for the Sociology of Family Life* (pp. 3–18). Basingstoke; New York: Palgrave Macmillan.

Dickerson, F. B. (1998). Strategies That Foster Empowerment. *Cognitive and Behavioral Practice, 5*(2), 255–275.

Didion, J. (2005). *The Year of Magical Thinking.* New York: Knopf.

Doka, K. J. (1989). *Disenfranchised Grief: Recognizing Hidden Sorrow.* Lexington: Lexington Books.

Doka, K. J. (2002). *Disenfranchised Grief: New Directions, Challenges and Strategies for Practice.* Champaign, IL: Research Press.

Duffy, M., & Yell, S. (2014). Mediated Public Emotion: Collective Grief and Australian Natural Disasters. In D. Lemmings & A. Brooks (Eds.), *Emotions and Social Change* (pp. 99–116). Oxford: Routledge.

Ethical Guidelines for Assisted Reproductive Technology (ART). (n.d.). Retrieved from https://www.nhmrc.gov.au/health-ethics/ethical-issues/assisted-reproductive-technology-.

Ettore, E. (2002). A Critical Look at the New Genetics: Conceptualizing the Links Between Reproduction, Gender and Bodies. *Critical Public Health, 12*(3), 237–250.

Festinger, L. A. (1954). A Theory of Social Comparison Processes. *Human Relations, 7*(2), 117–140.

Fingeld, D. L. (2000). Therapeutic Groups Online: The Good, the Bad, and the Unknown. *Issues in Mental Health Nursing, 21*(3), 241–255.

Finn, J. (1995). Computer-Based Self-Help Groups: A New Resource to Supplement Support Groups. *Social Work with Groups, 18*(1), 109–117.

Francis, L. A. (1997). Ideology and Interpersonal Emotion Management: Redefining Identity in Two Support Groups. *Social Psychology Quarterly, 60*(2), 153–171.

Frank, A. (1995). *The Wounded Storyteller: Body, Illness & Ethics.* Chicago: University of Chicago Press.

Frank, A. (2010). *Letting Stories Breathe: A Socio-Narratology*. Chicago: University of Chicago Press.

Friedan, B. (1963). *The Feminine Mystique*. New York: W.W. Norton and Co.

Frith, L., & Blyth, E. (2014). Assisted Reproductive Technology in the USA: Is More Regulation Needed? *Reproductive Biomedicine Online, 29*(4), 516–523.

Frost, L. (2016). Exploring the Concepts of Recognition and Shame for Social Work. *Journal of Social Work, 30*(4), 431–446.

Furedi, F. (2004a). *The Therapy Culture: Cultivating Vulnerability in an Uncertain Age*. London; New York: Routledge.

Furedi, F. (2004b). Reflections on the Medicalisation of Social Experience. *British Journal of Guidance & Counselling, 32*(3), 413–415.

Gengler, A. (2015). "He's Doing Fine": Hope Work and Emotional Threat Management Among Families of Seriously Ill Children. *Symbolic Interaction, 38*(4), 611–630.

Gerrity, D. A. (2001). Five Medical Treatment Stages of Infertility: Implications for Counselors. *Family Journal, 9*(2), 140–150.

Gibson, M. (2016). Youtube and Bereavement Vlogging: Emotional Exchange Between Strangers. *Journal of Sociology, 52*(4), 631–645.

Giddens, A. (1979). *Central Problems in Social Theory*. London: Macmillan.

Giddens, A. (1991). *Modernity and Self-Identity: Self and Society in the Late Modern Age*. Cambridge: Polity.

Giddens, A. (1992). *The Transformation of Intimacy: Sexuality, Love and Eroticism in Modern Societies*. Cambridge: Polity Press.

Greco, M., & Stenner, P. (2008). *Emotions: A Social Science Reader*. London: Routledge.

Greene, M. J. (2014). On the Inside Looking In: Methodological Insights and Challenges in Conducting Qualitative Insider Research. *The Qualitative Report, 19*(29), 1–13.

Greer, G. (1984). *Sex and Destiny: The Politics of Human Fertility*. New York: Harper and Row.

Greil, A. L. (1991). *Not Yet Pregnant: Infertile Couples in Contemporary America*. New Brunswick: Rutgers University Press.

Greil, A. L. (1997). Infertility and Psychological Distress: A Critical Review of the Literature. *Social Science & Medicine, 45*(11), 1679–1704.

Greil, A., McQuillan, J., & Slauson-Blevins, K. (2011). The Social Construction of Infertility. *Sociology Compass, 5*(8), 736–746.

Groos, N. (2005). The Detraditionalization of Intimacy Reconsidered. *Sociological Theory, 23*(3), 286–311.

Gubrium, J. F. (2005). Introduction: Narrative Environments and Social Problems. *Social Problems, 52*(4), 525–528.

Gubrium, J. F., & Holstein, J. A. (2000). The Self in a World of Going Concerns. *Symbolic Interaction, 23*(2), 95–115.

Gubrium, J. F., & Holstein, J. A. (2009). *Analyzing Narrative Reality*. Thousand Oaks, CA: Sage.

Hanna, E., & Gough, B. (2016). Emoting Infertility Online: A Qualitative Analysis of Men's Forum Posts. *Health, 20*(4), 363–382.

Hanna, E., & Gough, B. (2017). Men's Accounts of Infertility Within Their Intimate Partner Relationships: An Analysis of Online Forum Discussions. *Journal of Reproductive and Infant Psychology, 35*(2), 150–158.

Harkness, S. K., & Hitlin, S. (2014). Morality and the Emotions. In J. E. Stets & J. H. Turner (Eds.), *Handbook of the Sociology of Emotions* (Vol. II, pp. 451–471). Dordrecht, Netherlands: Springer.

Harris, S. R. (2015). *An Invitation to the Sociology of Emotions*. Abingdon; Oxford: Taylor & Francis.

Hart, V. A. (2002). Infertility and the Role of Psychotherapy. *Issues in Metal Health Nursing, 23*(1), 31–41.

Hart, M. (2015). Youth Intimacy on Tumblr: A Pilot Study. *Young, 23*(3), 193–207.

Hinton, L., Kurinczuk, J. J., & Ziebland, S. (2010). Infertility; Isolation and the Internet: A Qualitative Interview Study. *Patient Education and Counseling, 81*(3), 436–441.

Hitchens, C. (2012). *Mortality*. London: Atlantic Books.

Hochschild, A. R. (1979). Emotion Work, Feeling Rules, and Social Structure. *American Journal of Sociology, 85*(3), 551–575.

Hochschild, A. R. (1983). *The Managed Heart: Commercialization of Human Feeling*. Berkeley, CA: University of California Press.

Holmes, K. (2016). Talking About Mental Illness: Life Histories and Mental Health in Modern Australia. *Australian Historical Studies, 47*(1), 25–40.

Holstein, J. A., & Gubrium, J. F. (2000). *The Self We Live By: Narrative Identity in a Postmodern World*. New York: Oxford University Press.

House, J. S., & Kahn, R. L. (1985). Measures and Concepts of Social Support. In S. Cohen & S. L. Syme (Eds.), *Social Support and Health* (pp. 83–108). Orlando, FL: Academic Press.

Hoybye, M. T., Johansen, C., & Tjornhoj-Thomsen, T. (2005). Online Interaction: Effects of Storytelling in an Internet Breast Cancer Support Group. *Psycho-Oncology, 14*(3), 211–220.

Hughes, E. C. (1984). *The Sociological Eye*. New Brunswick, NJ: Transaction Books.

Humbyrd, C. (2009). Fair Trade International Surrogacy. *Bioethics, 9*(3), 111–118.

Hunt, S. J. (2017). *The Life Course: A Sociological Introduction*. London; New York: Palgrave Macmillan.

Illouz, E. (1997). Who Will Care for the Caretaker's Daughter? Toward a Sociology of Happiness in the Era of Reflexive Modernity. *Theory, Culture & Society, 14*(4), 31–66.

Illouz, E. (2003). *Oprah Winfrey and the Glamour of Misery*. New York: Columbia University Press.

Illouz, E. (2007). *Cold Intimacies: The Making of Emotional Capitalism*. Cambridge, UK: Polity Press.

Illouz, E. (2008). *Saving the Modern Soul: Therapy, Emotions, and the Culture of Self-Help*. Berkeley, CA: University of California Press.

Illouz, E., Gilon, D., & Shachak, M. (2014). Emotions and Cultural Theory. In J. E. Stets & J. H. Turner (Eds.), *Handbook of the Sociology of Emotions* (Vol. II, pp. 221–244). Dordrecht, Netherlands: Springer.

Inhorn, M., & van Balen, F. (2002). *Infertility Around the Globe: New Thinking on Childlessness, Gender, and Reproductive Technologies*. Berkeley: University of California Press.

Jaffe, J. (2017). Reproductive Trauma: Psychotherapy for Pregnancy Loss and Infertility Clients from a Reproductive Story Perspective. *Psychotherapy, 54*(4), 380–385.

Jasper, J. M. (2014). Constructing Indignation: Anger Dynamics in Protest Movements. *Emotion Review, 6*(3), 208–213.

Joinson, A. N. (2001). Self-Disclosure in Computer-Mediated Communication: The Role of Self-Awareness and Visual Anonymity. *European Journal of Social Psychology, 31*(2), 177–192.

Karp, D. (2001). *The Burden of Sympathy: How Families Cope with Mental Illness*. Oxford; New York: Oxford University Press.

Kawachi, I., & Berkman, L. F. (2001). Social Ties and Mental Health. *Journal of Urban Health, 78*(3), 458–467.

Lapidot-Lefler, N., & Barak, A. (2015). The Benign Online Disinhibition Effect: Could Situational Factors Induce Self-Disclosure and Prosocial Behaviors? *Cyberpsychology: Journal of Psychosocial Research on Cyberspace, 9*(2), Article 3, 1–19.

Leigh, J. (2016). *Avalanche: A Love Story*. Melbourne: Penguin Group Australia.

Lewis, C. S. (1961). *A Grief Observed*. London: Faber.

Lieberman, M. A., & Goldstein, B. A. (2006). Not All Negative Emotions Are Equal: The Role of Emotional Expression in Online Support Groups for Women with Breast Cancer. *Psycho-Oncology, 15*(2), 160–168.

Lively, K. J., & Weed, E. A. (2014). Emotion Management: Sociological Insight into What, How, Why, and to What End? *Emotion Review, 6*(3), 202–207.

Lourde, A. (1980). *The Cancer Journals*. San Francisco: Aunt Lute Books.

Lupton, D. (2012). 'Precious Cargo': Foetal Subjects, Risk and Reproductive Citizenship. *Critical Public Health, 22*(3), 329–340.

Lupton, D. (2013). *Risk*. London; New York: Routledge.

Lupton, D. (2015). *Digital Sociology*. Abingdon: Routledge.

Lupton, D. (2016). *The Quantified Self: A Sociology of Self-Tracking*. Cambridge: Polity.

Macaldowie, A., Lee, E., & Chambers, G. M. (2013). *Assisted Reproductive Technology in Australia and New Zealand 2013*. National Perinatal Epidemiology and Statistics Unit, the University of New South Wales. Retrieved from https://npesu.unsw.edu.au/sites/default/files/npesu/data_collection/Assisted%20reproductive%20technology%20in%20Australia%20and%20New%20Zealand%202013.pdf.

Malik, S. H., & Coulson, N. S. (2008a). Computer-Mediated Infertility Support Groups: An Exploratory Study of Online Experiences. *Patient Education and Counseling, 73*(1), 105–113.

Malik, S. H., & Coulson, N. S. (2008b). The Male Experience of Infertility: A Thematic Analysis of an Online Infertility Support Group Bulletin Board. *Journal of Reproductive and infant psychology, 26*(1), 18–30.

Malik, S. H., & Coulson, N. S. (2010). Coping with Infertility Online: An Examination of Self-Help Mechanisms in an Online Infertility Support Group. *Patient Education and Counseling, 81*(2), 315–318.

Matthews, R., & Matthews, A. M. (1986). Infertility and Involuntary Childlessness: Transition to Non-Parenthood. *Journal of Marriage and the Family, 48*(3), 641–649.

May, V. (2012). Narrative Analysis and Interpretive Phenomenological Analysis. In C. Seale (Ed.), *Researching Society and Culture* (pp. 441–458). *London: Sage*.

May, V. (2013). *Connecting Self to Society: Belonging in a Changing World*. Basingstoke: Palgrave Macmillan.

McEwan, I. (2007). *On Chesil Beach*. New York: Doubleday.

McKenna, K. Y. A., & Bargh, J. A. (2000). Plan 9 from Cyberspace: The Implications of the Internet for Personality and Social Psychology. *Personality and Social Psychology Review, 4*(1), 57–75.

Medew, J. (2016, November 14). IVF Clinics Caught Making False and Misleading Claims About Success Rates. *The Age*. Retrieved from http://www.theage.com.au/victoria/ivf-clinics-caught-making-false-and-misleading-claims-about-success-rates-20161114-gsooix.html.

Miller, J. K., & Gergen, K. J. (1998). Life on the Line: The Therapeutic Potentials of Computer-Mediated Conversation. *Journal of Marital and Family Therapy, 24*(2), 189–202.

Mo, P. K. H., & Coulson, N. S. (2014). Are Online Support Groups Always Beneficial? A Qualitative Exploration of the Empowering and Disempowering Processes of Participation Within HIV/AIDS-Related Online Support Groups. *International Journal of Nursing Studies, 51*(7), 983–993.

Newton, C. R., Sherrad, W., & Glavac, I. (1999). The Fertility Problem Inventory: Measuring Perceived Fertility Related Stress. *Fertility and Sterility, 72*(1), 54–62.

O'Reilly, A. (2010). *Twenty-First-Century Motherhood: Experience, Identity, Policy, Agency*. New York: Columbia University Press.

Parks, M. R., & Floyd, K. (1996). Making Friends in Cyberspace. *Journal of Communication, 46*(1), 80–97.

Patterson, W. (2002). Narrative Imaginings: The Liminal Zone in Narratives of Trauma. In W. Patterson (Ed.), *Strategic Narrative: New Perspectives on the Power of Personal and Cultural Stories* (pp. 71–88). Lanham, MD: Lexington Books.

Peng, L. (2013). Surrogate Mothers: An Exploration of the Empirical and the Normative. *American University Journal of Gender, Social Policy and Law, 21*(3), 555–582.

Pennebaker, J. W. (1997). Writing About Emotional Experiences as a Therapeutic Process. *Psychological Science, 8*(3), 162–166.

Pennebaker, J. W., & Evans, J. F. (2014). *Expressive Writing: Words that Heal*. Enumclaw, WA: Idyll Arbor.

Pennebaker, J. W., & Seagal, J. D. (1999). Forming a Story: The Health Benefits of Narrative. *Journal of Clinical Psychology, 55*(10), 1243–1254.

Pennebaker, J. W., & Smyth, J. (2016). *Opening Up by Writing It Down: The Healing Power of Expressive Writing*. New York: Guilford.

Petersen, A. (1996). Risk and the Regulated Self: The Discourse of Health Promotion as Politics of Uncertainty. *Australia and New Zealand Journal of Sociology, 31*(1), 44–57.

Petersen, A. (1997). Risk, Governance and the New Public Health. In A. Petersen & R. Bunton (Eds.), *Foucault, Health and Medicine* (pp. 189–206). London: Routledge.

Peterson, B. D., Newton, C. R., Rosen, K. H., & Skaggs, G. E. (2003). Examining Congruence Between Partners' Perceived Infertility-Related Stress and Its Relationship to Marital Adjustment and Depression in Infertile Couples. *Family Process, 42*(1), 59–70.

Rheingold, H. (1993). *The Virtual Community: Homesteading on the Electronic Frontier*. Reading, MA: Addison-Wesley.

Rich, A. (1977). *Of Woman Born: Motherhood as Institution*. London: Virago.

Richardson, L. (1990). Narrative and Sociology. *Journal of Contemporary Ethnography, 19*(1), 116–135.

Ricoeur, P. (1991). Life in Quest of Narrative (trans. D. Wood). In D. Wood (Ed.), *On Paul Ricoeur: Narrative and Interpretation* (pp. 20–33). London: Routledge.

Ridings, C., Gefen, D., & Arinze, B. (2002). Some Antecedents and Effects of Trust in Virtual Communities. *Journal of Strategic Information Systems, 11*(3), 271–295.

Ridings, C., Gefen, D., & Arinze, B. (2006). Psychological Barriers: Lurker and Poster Motivation and Behavior in Online Communities. *Communications of the Association for Information Systems, 18*, 329–355.

Riessman, C. K. (2001). Personal Troubles as Social Issues: A Narrative of Infertility in Context. In I. Shaw & N. Gould (Eds.), *Qualitative Research in Social Work* (pp. 73–83). London: Sage.

Saleebey, D. (1994). Culture, Theory, and Narrative: The Intersections of Meaning in Practice. *Social Work, 39*(4), 351–359.

Savitz-Smith, J. (2003). Couples Undergoing Fertility Treatment: Implications for Counselors. *The Family Journal, 11*(4), 383–386.

Schmidt, L., Bjørn, H., Christensena, U., & Boivinb, J. (2005). "Does Infertility Cause Marital Benefit?" An Epidemiological Study of 2250 Women and Men in Fertility Treatment. *Patient Education and Counseling, 59*(3), 244–251.

Shaw, B. R., Hawkins, R., Arora, N., McTavish, F., Pingree, S., & Gustafson, D. H. (2006). An Exploratory Study of Predictors of Participation in a Computer Support Group for Women with Breast Cancer. *CIN: Computers, Informatics, Nursing, 24*(1), 18–27.

Silva, J. (2013). *Coming Up Short: Working-Class Adulthood in an Age of Uncertainty*. New York: Oxford University Press.

Silverman, D. (2010). *Doing Qualitative Research*. London: Sage.

Singleton, A., Abeles, P., & Smith, I. C. (2016). Online Social Networking and Psychological Experiences: The Perceptions of Young People with Mental Health Difficulties. *Computers in Human Behavior, 61*(August), 394–403.

Slauson-Blevins, K. S., McQuillan, J., & Greil, A. L. (2013). Online and In-Person Health-Seeking for Infertility. *Social Science & Medicine, 99*(December), 110–115.

Solomon, D. H. (2016). Relational Turbulence Model. In C. R. Berger & M. E. Roloff (Eds.), *The International Encyclopaedia of Interpersonal Communication*. Hoboken, NJ: John Wiley & Sons, Inc.

Solomon, D. H., & Knobloch, L. K. (2004). A Model of Relational Turbulence: The Role of Intimacy, Relational Uncertainty, and Interference from Partners in Appraisals of Irritations. *Journal of Social and Personal Relationships, 21*(6), 795–816.

Staples, L. H. (1990). Powerful Ideas About Empowerment. *Administration in Social Work, 4*(2), 29–42.

Steuber, K. R., & Solomon, D. H. (2008). Relational Uncertainty, Partner Interference, and Infertility: A Qualitative Study of Discourse within Online Forums. *Journal of Social and Personal Relationships, 25*(5), 831–855.

Steuber, K. R., & Solomon, D. H. (2012). Relational Uncertainty, Partner Interference, and Privacy Boundary Turbulence: Explaining Spousal Discrepancies in Infertility Disclosures. *Journal of Social and Personal Relationships, 29*(1), 3–27.

Styron, W. (1990). *Darkness Visible: A Memoir of Madness*. New York: Random House.

Suler, J. (2004). The Online Disinhibition Effect. *CyberPsychology & Behavior, 7*(3), 321–326.

Symth, J. M., Stone, A. A., Hurewitz, A., & Kaell, A. (1999). Effects of Writing About Stressful Experiences on Symptom Reduction in Patients with Asthma or Rheumatoid Arthritis: A Randomized Trial. *Journal of the American Medical Association, 281*(14), 1304–1309.

Tanis, M. (2007). Online Social Support Groups. In A. N. Joinson, K. Y. A. McKenna, T. Postmes, & U.-D. Reips (Eds.), *The Oxford Handbook of Internet Psychology* (pp. 139–153). Oxford: Oxford University Press.

The Reproductive Technologies Council. (2016). Assisted Reproductive Technology Glossary. Retrieved from http://www.rtc.org.au/assisted-reproductive-technology-glossary/.

Thompson, C. M. (2002). *Fertile Ground: Feminists Theorize Infertility*. In M. Inhorn & F. van Balen (Eds.), *Infertility Around the Globe: New Thinking on Childlessness, Gender, and Reproductive Technologies* (pp. 52–78). California: University of California Press.

Throsby, K. (2004). *When IVF Fails: Feminism, Infertility and the Negotiation of Normality*. Hampshire: Palgrave Macmillan.

Turner, R. J., & Brown, R. L. (2012). Social Support and Mental Health. In T. L. Scheid & T. N. Brown (Eds.), *A Handbook for the Study of Mental Health: Social Contexts, Theories and Systems* (pp. 200–212). Cambridge: Cambridge University Press.

van Uden-Kraan, C. F., Drossaert, C. H. C., Taal, E., Seydel, E. R., & van Laar, M. A. F. (2008). Self-Reported Differences in Empowerment Between Lurkers and Posters in Online Patient Support Groups. *Journal of Medical Internet Research, 10*(2), e18.

Wallace, P. (1999). *The Psychology of the Internet*. Cambridge: Cambridge University Press.

Waller, V., Farquharson, K., & Dempsey, D. (2015). *Qualitative Social Research: Contemporary Methods for the Digital Age*. Los Angeles: Sage Publications.

Walter, T. (2007). Modern Grief, Postmodern Grief. *International Review of Sociology, 17*(1), 123–134.

White, M., & Dorman, S. M. (2001). Receiving Social Support Online: Implications for Health Education. *Health Education Research, 16*(6), 693–707.

Wilding, R. (2006). Virtual Intimacies? Families Communicating across Transnational Contexts. *Global Networks: A Journal of Transnational Affairs, 6*(2), 125–142.

Wilkinson, I., & Kleinman, A. (2016). *A Passion for Society: How We Think About Human Suffering*. Oakland, CA: University of California Press.

Woodward, K., & Woodward, S. (2009). *Why Feminism Still Matters: Feminism Lost and Found*. Basingstoke; New York: Palgrave Macmillan.

Wright, K. (2000). Computer-Mediated Social Support, Older Adults and Coping. *Journal of Communication, 50*(3), 100–118.

Wright, K. (2008). Theorizing Therapeutic Culture: Past Influences, Future Directions. *Journal of Sociology, 44*(4), 321–336.

Wright Mills, C. (1959). *The Sociological Imagination*. Oxford: Oxford University Press.

Wurtzel, E. (1994). *Prozac Nation: Young and Depressed in America*. Boston: Houghton Mifflin.

Yeatman, A. (2009). *Individualisation and the Delivery of Welfare Services.* New York: Palgrave Macmillan.

Zegers-Hochschild, F., Adamson, G. D., de Mouzon, J., Ishihara, O., Mansour, R., Nygren, K., et al. (2009). International Committee for Monitoring Assisted Reproductive Technology (ICMART) and the World Health Organization (WHO) Revised Glossary of ART Terminology. *Fertility and Sterility, 92*(5), 1520–1524.

Index

© The Author(s) 2019
P. Billett, A.-M. Sawyer, *Infertility and Intimacy in an Online Community*,
Palgrave Macmillan Studies in Family and Intimate Life,
https://doi.org/10.1057/978-1-137-44981-8